Do you have or think you have a hernia?

A step by step guide for patients to help them analyze their problem and seek an intelligent plan of treatment.

THE HERNIA SOLUTION

Myths · Facts · Answers

By James A. Bulen, M.D., F.A.C.S.
and
Charles F. Bridgman, Ph.D.

Edited by Matthew Midgett, B.A.

Published by Advanced Health Press

So teach us to number our days that we may get a heart of wisdom.

Psalms 90, Verse 12

Foreword

Drs. Bulen and Bridgman have produced an authoritative guide for patients suffering from a variety of hernial problems. I have been involved with this subject since the mid-1950's and know how concerned my patients have been with the innumerable details of the cause, treatment and results of hernia operations. Many answers to these concerns are clearly presented by the authors.

The use of short patient reports is helpful. We, as patients, will recognize quickly whether or not a given sequence of happenings in these reports fits our own symptom complex.

More than 500,000 operations for hernias are performed in the United States every year. I can imagine the relief given to many of these patients when reassured by the factual information presented in this fine guide.

Lloyd M. Nyhus, M.D., F.A.C.S., Drs. h.c.
Warren H. Cole Professor of Surgery
The University of Illinois
College of Medicine at Chicago

THE HERNIA SOLUTION

Myths · Facts · Answers

A Comprehensive Guide to Patient Care

By James A. Bulen, M.D.
and
Charles F. Bridgman, Ph. D.

Published by
Advanced Health Press
Suite 233-A
716 East Valley Parkway
Escondido, CA 92025-3097

Copyright © 1992 by James A. Bulen and Charles F. Bridgman.
First printing 1992

Library of Congress number 91-091955
Library of Congress Cataloging in Publication Data
Bulen, James A.; Bridgman, Charles F.
The Hernia Solution: Myths•Facts•Answer - 1st ed.
Hernias; Hernias abdominal wall
Includes index
RD621. B85 1991 LMWI 955 617.559
ISBN 0-9630114-4-8 Softcover $19.95
ISBN 0-9630114-5-6 Hardcover $24.95

Introduction

In the past few years, I became fascinated with the challenges and problems of hernia surgery. While working as a general surgeon, I had performed more than 2500 hernia operations. Recently, when the opportunity arose, I was pleased to dedicate my attention to hernia care. This has been a most rewarding experience. Attending national symposiums, I have been delighted to find other surgeons with the same interests and specialization.

While caring for my patients, I have been impressed by their thirst for knowledge about hernias. Initially a small pamphlet was produced, then a booklet, and finally this book. This is an attempt to respond to the patient's desire for education and instruction. Hopefully, this book will help you sail smoothly through the course of your hernia care.

The book describes a hernia for you in lay terminology. The more common varieties of hernias will be discussed, along with the appropriate treatment.

This is not a medical text. However, it is medically exacting enough to be used by medical students, physicians, and nurses who wish to help patients through their hernia care.

James A. Bulen, M.D., F.A.C.S.

Dedication

To my patients who have allowed me to care for them, and have stimulated me to understand their concerns and needs for communication.

To my wife, Gina Louise Bulen, Ph.D., J.D., who is my constant source of inspiration and encouragement.

To my office manager and friend, Aldine Osborne, who is everything a busy physician, or an anxious patient, could ask for.

JAB

Appreciation

Writing a book is not a solo project. Had it not been for the enthusiastic encouragement and support of so many, this book would have remained unwritten.

A tremendous amount of gratitude and affection goes to Dr. Lawrence Getz, M.D., F.A.C.S., for his many hours of both support *and* leadership in the operating room.

Special mention to Richard Kemp Massengill M.D., for his inspiration, and for challenging me to undertake this project.

It has been a special pleasure to work with my friend, Charles Bridgman, on this book. His skills with illustration and text revision have greatly enhanced this work.

Matthew Midgett, Editor, has applied his upbeat editorial skills to this manuscript from start to finish. Matthew, at all times, sees it from the patient's point of view.

A special thanks is given to San Diego Union Columnist Don Freeman, who cheerfully gives of his time to teach. His support and guidance were invaluable in the development of my writing skills.

Anesthesiologists have been very supportive as a group and I would, particularly, name a few, in alphabetical order: Donald Bernstein, M.D., Marc Gipsman, M.D., Marvin Levenson, M.D., Martin Mann, M.D., Deborah Mitchell, M.D., and David Slack, M.D.

Nurses have been instrumental in the development of the routines for care of my hernia patients. They have been involved in all aspects of the patient's care, contributing to the original evaluation of the patient's general health, the preparation for surgery, the maintenance of operating room equipment, the support in the operating room and recovery room, the making of house calls, and other generalized support all along the way.

I would like to thank a few of these nurses, once again in alphabetical order: Denise Bairesema, O.R.T., C.R.A., Evelyn Buensuceso, R.N., June Chelsvig, R.N., Ann E. Dechairo, R.N., M.S., Beverly Ervin, R.N., Virginia Field, R.N., B.A., Virginia Goheen, L.V.N., Glen Intermill, R.N., April Kasten, R.N., Phyllis Lawrence, R.N., Barbara Massey, R.N., Sharon Masterson, R.N., Barbara Muterspaw, C.O.R.T., Deborah Nelson, R.N., Shannon Perry, M.A., Linda Phillips, L.V.N., Vicki Vosefski, R.N., and Sally Weinhart, R.N., F.N.P.

To Palomar Medical Center and the support of their medical secretary, Carolyn Edwards, and staff librarian, Amanda Rathbun, for making all the medical literature about hernias published in the past three years available for my review.

Thanks to Mary Ellen Alton whose artistic skills and knowledge of PageMaker helped to coordinate the text and illustrations.

Lastly, to my son, James Jr., for sharing his computer with me. Jimmy has helped develop a spread sheet so that the care of all the hernia patients in my practice may be followed and analyzed. And, this same computer has made the production of this book so much easier.

JAB

Table of Contents

List of Illustrations

Notice — Disclaimer

This book is designed to provide information about the subject matter covered. It is sold with the understanding that the authors, illustrator and publisher are not engaging in the rendering of professional medical advice or services. This book is not intended to be an alternate to appropriate medical care.

The purpose of this book is to educate and entertain. The author-publisher shall have neither liability nor responsibility to any person or entity with respect to any loss or damage caused, or alleged to be caused, directly or indirectly by the information contained in this book.

If you do not wish to be bound by the above, you may return this book along with your sales receipt to the publisher within thirty days for a full refund.

Advanced Health Press
Suite 233-A
716 East Valley Parkway
Escondido, CA 92025-3097

Chapter One

Revolution In Hernia Surgery

There is a revolution going on! It is a revolution by surgeons who are quietly changing the way surgery is being performed on patients with hernias. The revolution has been joined by patients who are seeking educated information about their care; by insurance companies and health care facilities seeking to control costs; by statisticians conducting research on surgical procedures and carefully tracking the progress of patients for the most important reason of all — **results!**

Now this isn't a revolution with injuries and deaths. Rather it is a revolution with improved care and improved service — improved sharing of facts and figures. And who benefits *most* from all of this? *The patient.*

This book is about that revolution. It discusses the changes that are taking place as hernia surgery is re-evaluated and changed, with the patient as the ultimate beneficiary.

During the past 50 years, hernia surgery has been performed by general surgeons and by general practitioners. These dedicated physicians have maintained a general interest in medicine in all its facets, and have performed a myriad of services while also seeing and treating a relatively small number of patients with hernias. Now, greater specialization enhances hernia care.

Contemporary hernia techniques were developed during the past 100 years and were *gradually* improved upon until fairly recently. However, the attention of surgical trainees was not focused on the *hernia* patient. During the first year of exposure to surgery, a medical resident learned to perform a hernia operation and during the next few years dedicated himself or herself to learning how to treat and operate on "more exotic and challenging problems".

Recently, surgical training centers have begun to develop services which *specialize* in the treatment of hernias, and which require standardization of techniques and on results. An example of this is the Hernia Center in Down State New York Hospital, where specialization has produced superior results for the hernia patient.

Some physicians, having completed their surgical training, dedicate themselves almost exclusively to hernia repairs. Centers dedicated to hernia repair are developing across the United States and throughout the world. Seminars and research studies directed specifically to hernia problems are being given with increased frequency.

In the United States, federally-funded Medicare insurance has had a great impact on hernia surgery. Medicare and private insurance companies insist that hernia surgery be performed in out-patient centers whenever possible; hospitalization for hernia surgery has been almost eliminated. The hospital stay is reserved for the rare complex hernia or for the otherwise very ill patient who also has a hernia.

Insurance companies and Medicare frequently require prior notification and approval before surgery may be performed. For example, CMRI (California Medical Review Institute) reviews and authorizes all Medicare hernia surgery prior to its performance. Insurance companies increasingly practice similar pre-operative review and approval or denial.

Out-Patient Surgery Centers

Responding to this demand, out-patient surgery centers have opened throughout the United States and offer efficient, effective, qualified service. The surgery is performed in the morning and the patient is back home within a matter of a few hours.

Clearly, *out-patient* surgery benefits the hernia patient in several ways. The primary benefit is the great familiarity with the procedure by both the surgeon and the *entire* support staff.

In recent years, convalescent centers which specialize in the care of the post-operative patient have been developed. Often located near the surgery center, these convalescent facilities accept overnight admissions of patients who have had hernia surgery. They are dedicated to the care of patients who need nursing support, special diets, occasional pain control, and understanding — but not critical nursing care. These centers fill the void between home and hospital.

Home Health Care

Nursing service has also changed. Home health care nurses are now available for house calls. They visit the patient in the home, make post-operative visits, give nursing care, and assist the family in caring for the patient. Both patients and relatives benefit from the comfort and convenience of care at home.

New Developments

Surgeons have changed their techniques. "Interrupted" or single sutures, placed one at a time, frequently are being replaced by running sutures, which distribute the tension evenly throughout the suture line. Closure of hernia incisions can be performed with little or no tension on the suture line, improving post-operative comfort and "durability" of the repair.

New materials have been developed. Sutures, formerly of silk, cotton or other natural fibers, have been replaced by monofilamented sutures of synthetic materials, such as polypropylene. Synthetics in the form of mesh, sheets or patches have been developed which allow the reinforcement of incision repairs with materials that are well-tolerated by the patient. These have been a major contribution to the "hernia" revolution. They allow more predictable results and much greater patient comfort during recovery.

Advances in anesthesia have been valuable to the hernia revolution. The development of new techniques in general anesthesia administration allow the patient to go to sleep and recover quickly.

New medications for the control of nausea and other side effects have been very helpful. Long-duration local anesthesia has been developed during the past ten years. All of these factors have contributed greatly to the patient's comfort following surgery.

Post-operative pain relief has taken a giant step forward. New, stronger, oral pain medications are available for use. New devices are becoming available that allow patients to self-administer *intravenous* pain medication. This is known as "patient-controlled analgesia" (PCA).

Use of antibiotics has dramatically changed. Surgeons are no longer satisfied with a one to three percent post-operative infection rate. Now, antibiotics are given intravenously before surgery, or are placed in the incision during the operation, as surgeons strive for a *zero* percent infection rate.

Hospitals and surgery centers have created quality care committees to evaluate all complications on a regular basis. Statistics relative to complications, infections, and prolonged hospitalization are immediately available. These statistics, available through computerized follow-up, allow surgeons, institutions, and insurance companies, to analyze results — particularly surgical outcome. A major advantage of computerization is the immediate recognition of problems that can then be very quickly corrected.

Finally, patients have become more involved in their own care. Today, people are far more knowledgeable and better educated. Patients *want* to be better informed about their own health care, illness, and treatment. New patient information publications have played a major role in educating the public. Medical programs on television, and videos are available on selected subjects. These have served to inform the general public. A well-informed, cooperative patient is instrumental in a successful outcome.

So, that's what this book is about — a revolution in hernia surgery. It has happened in a very quiet way, but nonetheless has had a dramatic effect in improving the care and treatment of patients with hernias.

No book can answer *all* the possible questions about a medical topic, but we sincerely hope that this information will provide you with useful facts, handy tips, comfort and confidence.

Hopefully, the information in the following chapters will provide you with useful facts and answers and will lead you to the solution to the proper care of your hernia.

Chapter Two

An Ounce of Prevention

MYTH: If I Ignore It, Maybe It Will Go Away.

FACT: We All Grow Older, Most Hernias Grow Larger.

So you, or someone dear to you, has developed a hernia, or suspects that a hernia exists. Your first inclination may be to "fix it" without surgery, and purchase a truss.

Some patients avoid surgery until they have an emergency, such as incarceration. Others seek out information, visit their physicians, and arrange for elective repair.

Cautious and conscientious patients will also use exercise and dietary control to prevent recurrences.

Let's look at some of these "strategies" and consider the benefits of each.

Typical Patients

"Tiny", 6'7", 64 years old, was an old friend from prior successful surgical treatments. Grateful to the author, but low on finances, and without medical insurance coverage, he purchased a truss (which fit nicely) and waited for his 65th birthday.

"Oscar", 78 years old, rather feeble, deaf, and with moderate angina and markedly irregular heart rate, came in for evaluation and possible surgery. The author, concerned about Oscar's heart and general medical condition, was cautious and initially prescribed a truss. Fitted and refitted without successful control of the hernia, the truss was discarded and Oscar had his right inguinal hernia repaired, uneventfully. Well-pleased, Oscar returned one year later for repair of a new hernia on the opposite side.

Trusses

Trusses are frequently the first "treatment" a patient chooses. Unfortunately, they often do not work.

If you insist on trying a truss, you should be well informed about its use, cost, fitting and method of application. Don Baker, RPh(Registered Pharmacist), who owns a pharmacy which includes a large inventory of medical supplies was asked to discuss trusses. He noted that he frequently fits *and tailors* a large number of trusses, then went on:

"*The adder-head spring truss is the standard for control of an inguinal hernia. Circular in fashion, a perineal (leg) band is needed to hold the pad firmly over the inguinal canal.*

"*The hernia must be completely and easily reducible by the patient if the truss is to be worn.* [If the hernia is not fully reduced, then the pressure from the truss may cause strangulation.] *The truss must be applied in the morning before the patient arises, and must be worn throughout the day.*"

Application of Trusses: *"If the rupture is out,"* Don states, *"lie down and reduce the hernia, taking the palm of your hand and gently pushing the hernia upward and in. If necessary, you may cough to locate the exact position of the rupture opening.* "The truss should be applied while lying down (on your back)."

Types of Trusses:

Spring Trusses: *"Spring trusses",* Don continues, *"are made of spring steel covered with leather and require considerable expertise to bend and shape the truss to the individual*

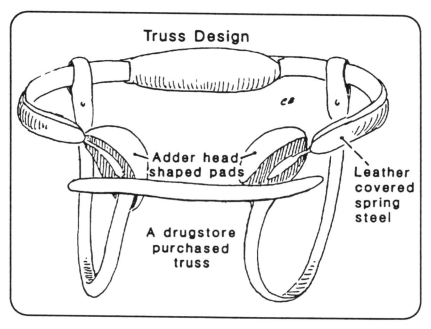

Figure 2-A

patient's body. Both the Double Spring Truss (see Figure 2-A) and the Single Spring Truss operate on the same mechanical principle, utilizing active pressure to retain the herniated tissue. If the patient has a bilateral hernia, then a double spring design is required. A single spring design may be used for a hernia on one side, or the patient may also wear a double spring design with a dummy pad on the non-involved side. A perineal (inner thigh) band can be used, depending on the configuration and need of the patient. These trusses sell for approximately $100."

Elastic Trusses: "These have the same therapeutic value as spring trusses," Don adds, "but are specifically suited for wear in bed. Perineal (thigh) straps are provided with this type of truss as an anchor to stabilize the elastic band. The therapeutic value of both the spring and elastic trusses is achieved by the action of pressure which controls the hernia by not allowing it to protrude."

Soft Pad Trusses: "These are much more comfortable and much easier to fit to the body. A hip measurement is taken to fit these, also, and they are worn for post-operative support or mild hernia support. They are made of cotton fabric with flat, oval hernia pads with flannel covers and with a cinching waistband in the back. These sell for about $40."

Hernia Prevention

Many hernias will appear, even though you are taking very good care of yourself. Congenital hernias can be prevented only by preselecting your parents. However, there are a fair number of hernias which appear because our bodies deteriorate. The important factors are discussed in depth in the chapter on recurrent inguinal hernias; there are a few items which deserve emphasis.

Patients should be within 10% to 15% of their optimal weight. Being overweight is an important cause of hernias, and their recurrences. And crash diets, with the resultant weight loss (and possible protein and vitamin loss) also contribute to hernia production.

Smoking and chronic coughing may be a frequent cause of hernias. Surprisingly, many smokers are not aware of their excessive coughing.

Maintenance of good nutrition is also important. Eating a diet with adequate supply of proteins is valuable. Additional vitamins are probably not needed when a patient enjoys the proper intake of foods. Supplemental vitamins should be considered, however, if there is a breach in the dietary intake.

Exercises

Exercise is important. Keeping active is not only good for your cardiopulmonary system (heart and lungs). It is also important to maintain good muscle strength of all the muscles in your body. It is not enough to just walk or swim. Some form of trunk twisting exercises are important, as this will help maintain the lateral trunk muscles where inguinal hernias occur. These muscles are illustrated in chapter 9. They are important in maintaining the strength or integrity of the abdominal wall and, hopefully, preventing hernias, such as direct inguinal hernias. No mention is made of sit-ups, which involve predominantly the rectus, or strap, muscles. These muscles are important, and sit-ups certainly may be a part of your exercise program.

The following exercises are given to you as examples. Only you and your doctor know if you may perform them with safety. Whatever you do, start with the easiest exercise first, and then progress *slowly*, changing exercises on a monthly, not a daily, basis.

Remember to alternate the exercises, doing them on one side, either singly or in a series, and then alternating to the other side.

1) Lying on your back, arms alongside (See Figure 2-B): Reach one hand toward the opposite hip. Allow that shoulder to raise from the mat, as you reach over. Pull the right lower chest toward the left hip, by contracting the abdominal muscles.

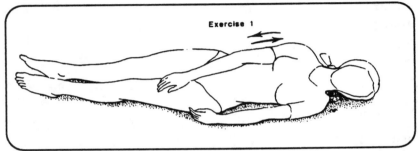

Exercise 1

Figure 2-B

2) Rotating flexing exercise from the lying position, hands behind your neck (See Figure 2-C): Draw up one thigh toward the opposite chest and reach with the knee toward the opposite elbow. Make progress by reaching further with the elbow. Try to relax the uninvolved elbow, and not push it against the mat.

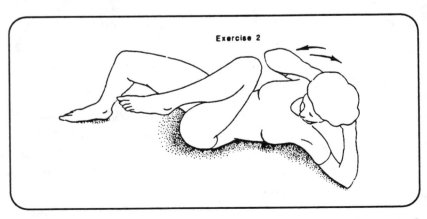

Exercise 2

Figure 2-C

3) Lying on your back, arms extended over your head:

A) Arm lead: Lead with your arm and shoulder, letting the chest turn as far as possible, then the pelvis and thigh may follow. The body may roll over partially or completely, but the rotation of the trunk is the most important action, as this strengthens the lateral abdominal muscles (See Figure 2-D, exercise, 3-A).

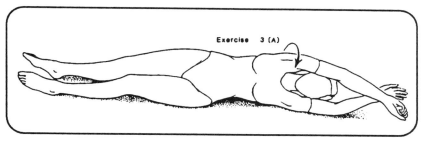

Figure 2-D

B) Pelvic lead: Initiate the roll with the pelvis, letting the arm and thigh lag behind (See Figure 2-E, exercise 3-B).

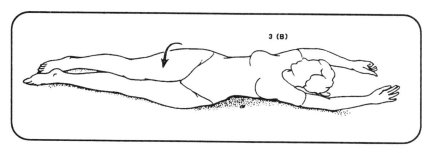

Figure 2-E

C) **Leg lead:** Start with the leg. The shoulders should remain on the mat as long as possible. The leg is allowed to rotate inward to emphasize the rotation of the trunk (See Figure 2-F, exercise 3-C).

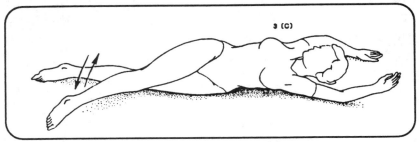

Figure 2-F

4) **Lateral exercises.** Flex your hip and knees which are on the mat. This will give your body stability during this exercise. (See Figure 2-G).

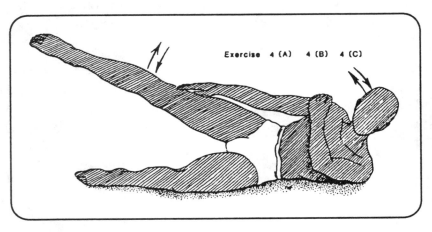

Figure 2-G

A) Raise your upper leg in line with the trunk. Lower slowly and repeat.

B) Raise your head off the mat, touching the ear to (or toward) the shoulder. Lower slowly and repeat.

C) Combine the leg and head lifts. Maintain alignment with the head and extremities with the trunk (do not allow either segment to flex or rotate).

5) **Lying on your back, arms comfortably extended for stability** (See Figure 2-H). Flex one thigh to a right angle from the trunk, then rotate the pelvis and touch toe to the floor on the opposite side at hip level. Return to the vertical, then lower thigh to mat.

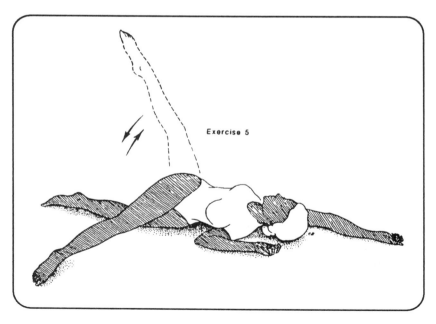

Exercise 5

Figure 2-H

During this exercise, remember to keep your chest as flat on the mat as possible. This may be easier to perform at first by touching the floor with the toe at the knee level, instead of the hip level. This exercise is also excellent for mobilizing the lower back.

Elective Repair

After it has been established that you have a hernia, and it has been determined that the appropriate mode of treatment is surgical, take time to select a surgeon, and a time and place for the repair. This is called an elective repair and this approach has a minimum of accompanying problems. Do not be trapped by a sudden situation, in which the hernia becomes incarcerated and has to be treated as an emergency. Then, you will give up the privilege of selecting the time and situation which will give you an optimal result. You may have a cold, or otherwise not be in an optimal state of health. You may have just eaten. (A full stomach means you will have to wait for six hours before it is safe to take a general anesthetic). You may have a trip planned the following week that you will have to postpone.

Prevention of Recurrence — Use of Prostheses

Synthetic materials (prostheses) have been used successfully to repair wounds for over thirty years. The material may be in the form of a mesh (Marlex®, or Mersilene®), or as a sheet (Gore-tex®, Dexon® and Vicryl®). These materials all have individual characteristics and advantages. Each material has its own advocates. Some, like Gore-tex®, are smooth surfaced, and are particularly valuable when a smooth face should be applied to the surrounding tissues. The materials are sewn into place by using sutures of the same synthetic material.

Graft rejection, or infection, is a source of great concern to all surgeons. This should be balanced against the risk of recurrence. The availability of antibiotics, with the subsequent fall in infection rates, has allowed the use of prosthetic materials to become commonplace.

Prevention of Infection

Although strict sterile technique is used, many surgeons administer antibiotics as well. These may be given intravenously, just prior to surgery, or may be placed in the operative site in the form of a solution or powder. Currently, infection rates after surgery are two to three percent. Recently published series using antibiotics reveal an infection rate of less than one percent. These excellent statistics are obtained when all of the patients are operated on under ideal circumstances.

Selection of Your Surgeon

It is important to select a physician who is well trained in surgery, preferably one who has performed a significant number of hernia surgeries, or in fact specializes in hernia repair. Find one who is interested in *your welfare*, and *his or her results*.

The Physician's Office

The physician's office and staff should be *available* to you. They should be ready and able to answer your questions during the day, and the *doctor or his associate should be available at any hour if a problem should arise.*

Costs are important and should be considered after quality. The doctor's office should be ready to explain their fees and to help you with your insurance billing and paperwork. Many offices now provide full billing services, arrangements for insurance authorizations, second opinions, and scheduling of home nursing visits at no extra cost to you.

Your relationship with the physician and his office staff is important. They should be friendly and should give you a feeling of peace of mind that relieves you of the administrative details which accompany your surgery. *Your surgeon and his office staff should be able, amiable and available.*

Conclusion

Some hernias are not "preventable". Others can be prevented by proper weight control, exercise, and other good health practices.

Many people consider the use of a truss as a first "treatment" for a hernia. Although they have some limited usefulness, trusses are generally an inadequate method of treatment. Hernia repair surgery is most often the treatment of choice. It is also preferable to have an "elective repair" when the time, location, and choice of surgeon can be determined by the patient. Some people avoid surgery and end up in an emergency situation which subjects them to greatly increased risk. **Don't let this happen to you.**

SOLUTION: If you have, or suspect you have a hernia, obtain medical consultation. Your fears will be allayed and you will then be in a position to make an informed decision.

Chapter Three

Inguinal Hernias In Infants and Children

An inguinal (in-gwen-al) hernia in an infant or child can be a life-threatening condition. Although the anatomy of a child's inguinal hernia is very similar to that of an indirect inguinal hernia in an adult, the surgical repair technique and the care of the patient differ greatly. The technique of repair for an infant will be discussed briefly.

A Typical Patient

"Eric" was 14 months old. Still breast feeding, he recently became "fussy" during the day, and his behavior didn't improve after eating. In fact, he didn't seem hungry.

A bulge had been noticed in his right groin when he was about 12 months old, and it now seemed to be enlarging.

Upon professional medical examination, the bulge was determined to be a hernia that extended along the groin into the upper part of his scrotum. It was approximately two finger-widths in size, tense and slightly tender. The hernia could not be pressed back into the abdomen (or "reduced") using firm pressure.

These symptoms indicated a very serious condition. Eric was scheduled for surgery immediately. The hernia was surgically opened and its contents evaluated. It was discovered that a tiny loop of intestine had been forced into the hernia sac. Fortunately, the intestine was healthy and after proper repositioning, no additional surgery, except repair of the hernia, was necessary.

The day following surgery, Eric felt much better and began nursing again. With his regular diet restored, he was released to home just two days after surgery.

Understandably, Eric's parents and grandparents were relieved. When his grandfather asked about the cause of the hernia, it was explained that it might very well have been an inherited trait. "Not from me," he retorted, "the boy's mother was adopted!"

We use this example because it provides a fairly typical scenario of an inguinal hernia in a small child. It also has a happy ending; fortunately, this is usually the case.

The Incidence of Inguinal Hernia

Inguinal hernias will occur in approximately 3.5% to 5% of all full-term newborns and are far more common among males with a ratio of nine to one.

Premature infants with low birth rate have up to 40% to 50% incidence of inguinal hernia.

Approximately 15% of those newborns with hernias will have hernias bilaterally (on both sides).

Embryonic Development of the Inguinal Area

The embryo first develops a testicle (or ovary) in the trunk, close to the kidney. By ten weeks this testicle or ovary begins to shift from the trunk into the lower abdomen, carrying its associated blood vessels with it. During normal development, each ovary travels into the pelvis and the testicles eventually leave the pelvic area and travel through the abdominal wall into the groin and on into the scrotum (See Figures 3-A and 3-B).

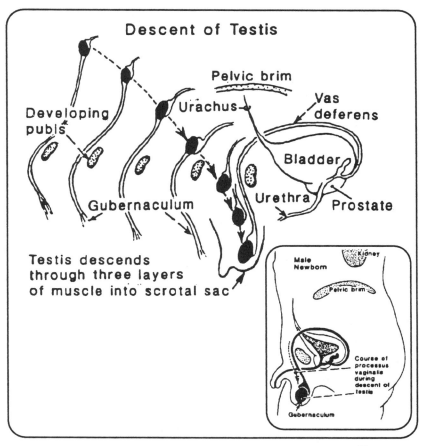

Figure 3-A

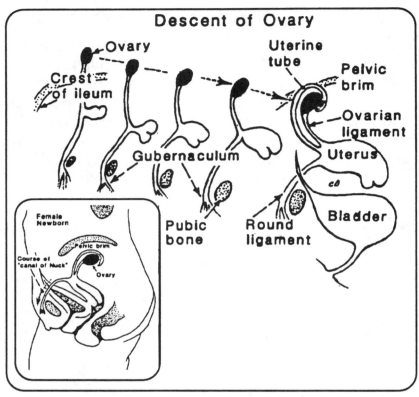

Figure 3-B

At about two months development in the fetus, the inner lining of the abdominal wall begins to close in the groin with a resulting bulge which eventually extends down into the scrotum in the male and the labia in the female. This extension is called a "processus vaginalis" in males, the "canal of Nuck" in the female. Later the testicles follow the path of the processus vaginalis into the scrotum. In both the male and the female the open channel may persist past its usefulness. In about 60% of normal infants at birth this may appear as a delicate, potentially open area extending from the abdomen into the groin.

In a small number of newborns, estimated at 5 %, the processus vaginalis (in the male) or the canal of Nuck (in the female) is enlarged. This enlargement is an inguinal hernia.

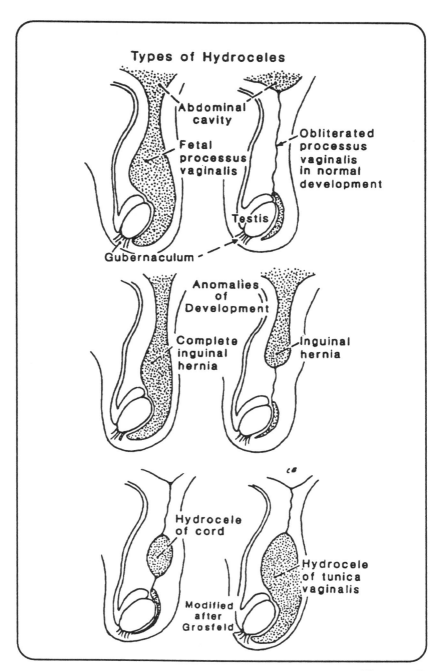

Types of Hydroceles

Abdominal cavity

Fetal processus vaginalis

Obliterated processus vaginalis in normal development

Testis

Gubernaculum

Anomalies of Development

Complete inguinal hernia

Inguinal hernia

Hydrocele of cord

Hydrocele of tunica vaginalis

Modified after Grosfeld

Figure 3-C

In males, it is *complete* if it extends all the way down the canal to the testicle, *incomplete* when it extends only part way. Figure 3-C shows the open processus in the male, and demonstrates the common anatomy shared by hernias and hydroceles.

Diagnosis of an Inguinal Hernia in an Infant

A "lump" in the groin of a child is a common problem presented to physicians. The history of its onset, its persistence and its exact location are critical to an accurate diagnosis. Parents should not be shy about examining this area; their description may be invaluable to the proper diagnosis of an inguinal hernia.

The lump, if it is a hernia, may become more prominent when the child cries or moves about vigorously.

It often disappears completely when the child is relaxed. The lump typically first appears at the inner portion of the groin area and may extend into the scrotal sac. In females, the lump may appear in the same area and may travel toward or into the labia.

Other "lumps" may be mistaken for an inguinal hernia in the male.

A condition known as a "hydrocele" may occur in the scrotum and is sometimes assumed by concerned parents to be a hernia.

Unlike an inguinal hernia, the hydrocele always stays in the scrotum. It does not change in size when the child cries or strains. It does not decrease in size when gentle pressure is applied on the scrotum toward the groin.

It is important to differentiate a hydrocele from an inguinal hernia, for the hydrocele usually disappears spontaneously and surgical treatment is *not* needed.

Other conditions that may imitate an inguinal hernia are relatively rare, but include enlarged or infected lymph nodes, a *femoral* hernia (see Chapter Six), an undescended testicle, an abscess, cystic enlargement of lymph tissue, and even a soft tissue tumor, such as a lipoma.

Obviously, accurate, timely diagnosis is essential to the child's health and well-being.

The Premature Infant

Advances in medical care of premature infants have resulted in a high survival rate. These same infants have an increased incidence of inguinal hernias. Complications, such as incarceration, strangulation, and gangrene of the testicle, are twice as frequent for these premature infants. These infants have immature development of their heart and lungs and the regulatory mechanisms of these systems as well. Therefore, care of the premature infant requires increased caution. Any surgical procedure required for a premature infant is usually delayed until just prior to release from the neonatal unit. Even then, the surgeon and anesthesiologist must exercise great caution during a surgical procedure. In the neonatal unit, every effort is made to reduce any hernia which protrudes.

Management of an Inguinal Hernia in a Premature Infant

If the hernia protrudes and requires surgery during the first two months after discharge from the neonatal unit, the infant is usually hospitalized again post-operatively to guard against complications from its weaker heart or lung regulatory mechanisms.

Management of an Inguinal Hernia in a Full-Term Infant

A full-term infant, without previous problems with breathing or heart rate, may be safely treated as an outpatient. With appropriate anesthetic and surgical precautions, early repair is accomplished with few complications and virtually zero mortality.

The high risk of incarceration and its associated complications in the pediatric age group makes the presence of an inguinal hernia an indication for surgical repair soon after diagnosis is made. All full-term infants and older children, without other illnesses, are treated as outpatients. Outpatient hernia surgery for children has been safe, effective, and well-tolerated for the past twenty years. The use of an outpatient surgical facility reduces cost to the patient's family, limits separation of child from parent, and reduces the psychological trauma to all concerned.

Description of a Typical Infant Hernia Repair

If the child is younger than six months of age, his or her extremities are wrapped and kept warm with a non-electrical heating device. All children receive careful monitoring of temperature, pulse, EKG, and tissue oxygen levels during the procedure.

The patient is given a general anesthetic, using a humidified anesthetic agent, and a breathing tube is inserted.

The patient is prepared for surgery and a tiny skin incision is made in the crease over the affected groin. Bleeding is almost non-existent and is easily controlled. The hernia sac is opened and the contents replaced into the abdomen. The sac is then tied at its origin and, usually, the rest of the sac wall is removed.

The incision is closed and absorbable sutures are placed under the surface of the skin, so that they will not have to be removed later. The wound is then dressed with a waterproof dressing.

Should The Opposite Side Be Explored at that Time?

Some physicians recommend exploration of the opposite side in an infant less than one year of age, because later re-operation for a second hernia is necessary in about 40% of these infants. After one year of age, only 11% will develop a hernia on the opposite side.

The exploration of a second side, after a hernia repair, takes an additional 20 minutes and can be pursued with very little risk if the operation and anesthetic are proceeding without difficulty.

Therefore, for a healthy child of less than one year of age, exploration of the opposite side should be considered and discussed with the surgeon before surgery is performed.

Management of an Absent Testicle

Sometimes, the testicle fails to descend into the scrotum. This is often associated with a hernia, and therefore should be discussed at this time. If the hernia is present, the two conditions should be treated at the same time. If there is no associated hernia, the *undescended* testicle should be explored for and treated (hopefully brought into a normal position in the scrotum) by one year of age.

Summary

It is frequently upsetting to parents when their infant or young child has a hernia.

Inguinal hernias occur in a small number of newborns and are more common among male infants. The incidence rises dramatically among premature babies.

A lump in the groin is the most frequent presenting symptom of an inguinal hernia in an infant or child. However, other medical conditions may be mistaken for a hernia and need to be differentiated from it. Hernia surgery in the healthy, full-term infant is a generally safe and straightforward outpatient procedure. It is always advisable to plan the surgery and perform it when the infant is healthy. Inguinal hernias in infants are prone to incarcerate and emergency repair is accompanied by increased risk.

Advances in medical care have resulted in the increased survival rate of many premature babies. Such infants are weaker at birth and surgery should be delayed if possible until they are more fully developed. The rate of complications is greater in premature infants.

About 40% of infants under the age of one with an inguinal hernia will develop a hernia on the opposite side. Therefore, some physicians recommend exploration of the opposite side during the initial hernia repair. Such exploration takes little time and poses little risk if the operation is proceeding smoothly.

Inguinal hernias in infants and children can be very serious and should not be neglected. Make sure your child receives attention as indicated by the presentation and symptoms.

Chapter Four

Inguinal Hernias in Adults

An inguinal (in-gwen-al) hernia is the most frequently occurring type of hernia. In fact, surgery to correct an inguinal hernia is among the most frequently performed and successful of all surgeries today. Medical practices specializing in hernia treatments report that approximately 90% of their patients come to them with this form of hernia.

The good news about inguinal hernia is this: It is relatively easy to diagnose and treat, and is generally *permanently* resolved with surgery.

Although quite specific in its characteristics, the inguinal hernia does share some traits with all hernias.

Some Typical Patients

"Roger", 58, an aviation engineer, had been noting an increasing bulge and an aching sensation in his left groin. His wife was worried and repeatedly asked him to see his doctor. Roger was also worried about the bulge, but was more concerned about his heart, since he was experiencing episodes of sharp pain in the "pit of his stomach". These pains, when evaluated in detail, often occurred when the bulge was largest, and the pain was occasionally accompanied by nausea and lower abdominal cramps.

In spite of these increasing symptoms, Roger continued to work and lead an active life. Finally, he experienced an attack of the previously experienced symptoms, plus vomiting. Instead of going to work that morning, he reported to his family physician and was referred to a hernia specialist, re-examined, and admitted directly to the hospital. He was operated on as an emergency that afternoon, after evaluating and "clearing" the status of his heart. He was found to have a large congenital inguinal hernia sac which contained loops of small intestine. There was inflammation of the loops of intestine, as well as inflammation of the hernia sac. The hernia was repaired after the intestine loops were examined and replaced into the abdomen. Roger had considerable abdominal discomfort and nausea the first 24 hours and was treated with intravenous fluids and "nothing by mouth". On the second post-operative day, his bowel function returned. Roger felt quite well again and was released to home care. He returned to work the following week, feeling better than he had during the entire past year.

"Jeanne", 67, a retired secretary, had "had a bad year". She had suffered an auto accident with knee, shoulder and back injuries. She had also noted an intermittent bulge in her right groin, but this was not particularly painful, compared to her other problems. She was seen by a hernia specialist in June, and was noted to have a small right inguinal hernia. In July, she had knee surgery. By November, she was beginning to notice the hernia more and her other injuries less. Jeanne had a right inguinal hernia repair, under local anesthesia, at an outpatient surgical center. She was back home in about four hours. She returned to an active life that first week.

"Mark", 28, a baker, noted a right groin lump after he lifted a heavy sack of flour. He felt some discomfort when it protruded, but he noted a relief from pain when he rested at night. He notified his employer of the bulge and pain, and was referred for care. He continued to work and, on occasion, would press the hernia back into place when it bulged. After approval from his employer's insurance company was obtained, the hernia was repaired. Like Jeanne, Mark's surgery was performed in an outpatient center. Mark had some swelling and discomfort in his wound the first two weeks, but spent most of his waking hours fixing things in and around the house. He returned to work after two weeks. At that time he was restricted to lifting 50 pounds, but after another two weeks began to lift without reservation.

"Allen", 79, a retired school principal, lived in an independent living facility adjacent to the nursing home where his wife was a resident. Allen had suffered a severe stroke twelve years earlier. At that time, he lost the ability to speak and was temporarily paralyzed on one side. Allen had a moderate-sized inguinal hernia which was bothering him. Fiercely independent in spite of his difficulties, he requested surgical repair. The hernia was repaired in the outpatient facility and he stayed overnight, at his facility, in an area where the nurses could visit him if needed. He never asked for help. He did take pain pills twice. He returned to his own apartment the following day.

"Roger", "Jeanne", "Mark" and "Allen" represent typical patients with inguinal hernias. All were quite concerned about their hernias and the surgery. After the surgery they were relieved and pleased.

Roger waited too long before asking for help. His hospitalization and discomfort could have been avoided had he obtained medical and surgical help earlier.

General Information About Hernias

A hernia is an abnormal bulge or protrusion of soft tissue in a body cavity that forces its way (or is forced by other pressures) through or between muscles.

Nearly always, this protrusion occurs at a site where the muscle wall of that cavity is weakened for some reason: physical damage to the wall, aging of the muscle tissue, or a hereditary predisposition to the hernia all may be contributing factors.

Typically, the protruded soft tissue forms a sac-like bulge that may also contain portions of organs, such as a loop of intestine.

If the hernia protrusion and its related "sac" can be easily returned through the muscle wall back into its original body cavity, the hernia is said to be "reducible". If the hernia is not *easily* returned, or if return is actually impossible, then it is considered "non-reducible" or "incarcerated". If the hernia becomes incarcerated, the patient may require emergency care.

Whenever a bulge cannot be easily pressed back or returned *and* there is simultaneous abdominal pain, emergency care must be received *immediately*.

Inguinal Hernia

An inguinal hernia is located at either the left or right groin area (where the abdomen and thigh meet). An inguinal hernia occurs commonly in males and occasionally in females. The increased incidence of occurrence in males is related to the anatomical structures associated with the testicle.

Hernias of the groin are of two types:

1. An *indirect* or *congenital* inguinal hernia protrudes down from the abdomen along the *inguinal canal*.

2. A *direct, or acquired* inguinal hernia occurs when abdominal organs push through a defect in the groin muscles of the *abdominal wall*.

Indirect (Congenital) Hernia

In the male fetus, each testicle migrates from a pelvic position within the abdomen, passes through the muscles of the abdominal wall and descends into the scrotum. The blood supply to the testicles and the vas deferens ("cord") follows this migration.

The normal "defect" or opening in the abdominal wall through which the testicle passes usually heals itself following completion of the migration. In some males this defect may remain, although it may not be noticeable until some time later

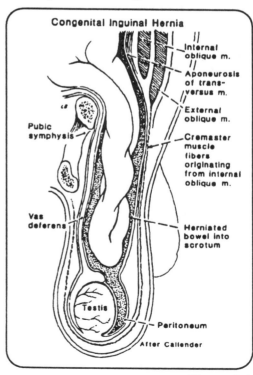

Figure 4-A

in life. These circumstances lead to a condition known as congenital (or inherited) indirect hernia.

Although congenital indirect hernias are most frequently found in children, adult patients may also present with this type of hernia late in life, even into the "senior" years. Congenital hernias are discussed in detail in Chapter Three, Inguinal Hernias in Infants and Children.

Direct Hernia

A direct inguinal hernia differs from a congenital inguinal hernia in its anatomical origin in the floor of the inguinal canal. The weakness in the floor of the inguinal canal usually becomes evident later in life, often after age 40. Remember, *indirect* inguinal hernias are due to an acquired "wear and tear" weakness in the abdominal wall. The connective tissue (fascia) gives way, allowing the hernia to develop. A *direct* inguinal hernia usually does not become as large as an indirect inguinal hernia and does not extend into the scrotum.

Factors which contribute to the development of a *direct* inguinal hernia include:

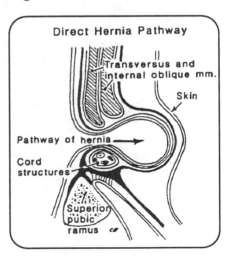

1) Muscle weakness which occurs with age, poor diet, significant changes in weight, and failure to exercise.

2) Stress on the abdominal wall as experienced with lifting or a sudden vigorous act.

3) Degeneration of the connective tissue forming the floor of the inguinal canal.

Figure 4-B

4) Pressure on the area from straining because of other physical problems. Examples often include chronic bronchitis or an acute respiratory infection with coughing, chronic asthma or other chronic lung disease, constipation and urinary outlet resistance (difficulty in urinating).

These factors are discussed in greater detail in the Chapter Five, Recurrent Inguinal Hernias.

Anatomy of the Inguinal Canal

The inguinal canal is a natural opening through the three layers of muscle at the lower portion of the lateral abdominal wall. The canal is approximately three inches long. Figure 4-C shows the external oblique muscle and fascia, the outer of those muscles.

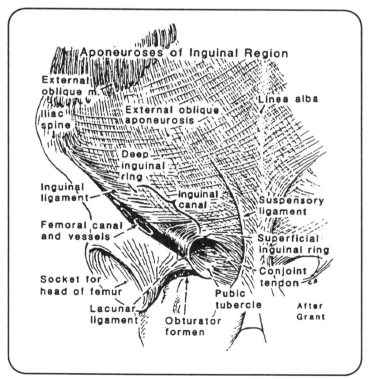

Figure 4-C

In the male, the testicles pass along the inguinal canal descending to the scrotum during fetal development. In the female, a ligament makes a similar descent through the canal into the groin area.

In both men and women, a sac-like extension of the tissue lining of the abdomen may extend along the inguinal canal. This is called an inguinal hernia. If the sac, or hernia, continues along the entire canal, it is called a *complete* inguinal hernia. If the sac appears *only* in the immediate area of a man's testicle, it is called a hydrocele. If the sac has forced its way along the vas deferens, it is known as a hydrocele of the cord. Figure 4-D demonstrates these relationships.

Although a hydrocele and an indirect (along the inguinal canal) inguinal hernia are related by their embryonic origin, they are treated separately according to their needs. Hydroceles that do not grow worse, seldom require surgical treatment, as they tend to resolve with time.

Most often, the patient does not give a history of a sudden, vigorous act resulting in a hernia. More commonly, the patient notices the gradual onset of discomfort and a bulge in the groin. Many patients are unaware that they have a direct inguinal hernia until a routine physical examination has been performed.

Diagnosis of an Inguinal Hernia

As with all medical conditions, effective treatment of hernias require early, accurate diagnosis.

Many patients discover hernias themselves, as a lump or larger bulge. Still others are surprised to learn of a hernia when it is found during a routine examination.

Either way, it takes an experienced physician to positively identify the type of hernia involved and recommend effective treatment.

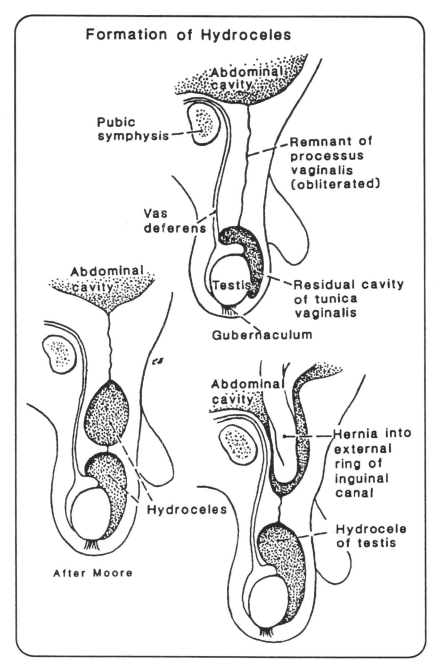

Formation of Hydroceles

Abdominal cavity

Pubic symphysis

Remnant of processus vaginalis (obliterated)

Vas deferens

Abdominal cavity

Testis

Residual cavity of tunica vaginalis

Gubernaculum

Abdominal cavity

Hernia into external ring of inguinal canal

Hydroceles

Hydrocele of testis

After Moore

Figure 4-D

An inguinal hernia should be diagnosed with the patient standing in front of the physician. The uninvolved side is examined first to establish the "norm" in that patient. If the patient is a male, the scrotum is moved to well below its junction with the abdominal wall and the physician's finger is brought behind the cord. In females, and in some males, the examination may be confined to the region of the inguinal canal. The physician simply feels portions of the inguinal canal with his finger-

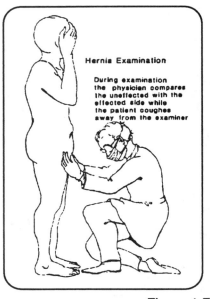

Hernia Examination

During examination the physician compares the unaffected with the affected side while the patient coughes away from the examiner

Figure 4-E

tips while the patient strains and/or coughs. An *indirect* hernia may be differentiated from a *direct* by the location of the bulge.

Some patients may experience pain in the inguinal canal for reasons other than a hernia. They may have "referred" or neighboring pain from other organs, such as the prostate or the bladder. Or, they may have an inflammatory problem of their cord structures or a recently injured muscle from a sudden vigorous act. None of these conditions indicate the presence of a hernia. **A diagnosis of an inguinal hernia is not made until the examiner feels a bulge. If there is no bulge, there is no hernia.**

Treatment of an Inguinal Hernia

The treatment of choice for an inguinal hernia is surgery. The use of new surgical techniques, synthetic mesh, local anesthetic (epidural anesthetic or a light general anesthetic), and the availability of outpatient facilities have combined to improve results and reduce recovery time. This is well supported by the medical literature in the United States and internationally, as well. A perspective on this problem is gained by reviewing the literature from Third-World countries, where hernia surgery is most frequently performed on an emergency basis, with a marked increase in complications, and even death. Stanley Berliner, M.D., evaluated 1,184 groin operations and reviewed the indications for surgery. Dr. Berliner stated, "*Surgery is needed for all femoral hernias and indirect hernias to prevent incarceration and strangulation. Direct inguinal hernias are also treated with surgery, with the exception of a small, direct hernia that is not enlarging or symptomatic.*"

When Should the Hernia Be Repaired?

The best time to have surgery is when you're feeling *well*. **Hernia surgery, if performed as an emergency, is followed by a twenty-fold increase in the rate of complication.** Naturally, emergency surgery will be performed immediately if the hernia becomes incarcerated or strangulated. Frequently, an inguinal hernia will remain small and asymptomatic. Then, it seems wise to plan the repair for a period in your life when you can take a week without the demands of work or travel. Most hernias are scheduled and repaired electively (at a time convenient to you, your family, and your doctor). But don't wait too long, for the hernia usually enlarges and, of course, you grow older.

Many surgeons are surprised as they review their patients' statistics and the patients' ages. In a recent series, over half of the patients with inguinal hernia repairs are over sixty years of age, and fully one-third of these are in their eighties. Hernia surgeons in New Jersey reported an uneventful repair of an inguinal hernia on a man 106 years old!

Author's Note: During a recent hernia seminar in Florida, a patient from New York was presented. Looking more like a patient from a third world country, he had an inguinal hernia which filled his scrotum, extending to six inches below his knees! All but the first and last few inches of his small and large intestine were in the hernia. Fortunately, he was not living in a Third World countries, and through the heroic efforts of modern medicine, the defect was safely repaired.

About Incarceration

An incarcerated hernia is, by definition, simply a hernia which cannot be "reduced" or moved back into proper position with gentle pressure.

When a hernia is incarcerated, pressure usually increases within the sac. This internal pressure then interferes with blood supply to the sac and its contents. This creates a vicious cycle of increasing pressure and decreasing blood flow.

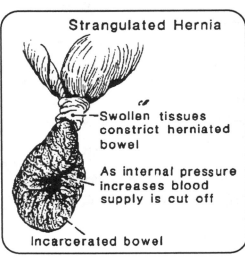

Strangulated Hernia

—Swollen tissues constrict herniated bowel

As internal pressure increases blood supply is cut off

Incarcerated bowel

Figure 4-F

If the flow of blood normally supplied to the contents of the sac (especially intestines) is obstructed, the contents become "strangulated". Progressive decrease in oxygen delivery (via blood circulation) to the hernia sac contents can result in gangrene, or tissue death. This is a life-threatening condition requiring immediate medical intervention.

The inability to reduce a hernia, of itself, is not necessarily an emergency. However, strangulation of bowel within the hernia creates a true surgical emergency and one that must be treated as soon as the diagnosis is made.

Any vigorous attempt by the surgeon to reduce an incarcerated hernia must be tempered with the awareness of two possible complications. First, the hernia may be "reduced en masse", that is, the hernia, *with sac intact*, is pushed back into the abdomen. Although the bulge is no longer obvious externally, the sac still exists, and the contents of the sac are still trapped within the sac and may undergo further deterioration or gangrenous changes. Therefore, following reduction of any incarcerated hernia, the patient must be carefully observed for signs of *continuing* intestinal obstruction or injury.

The second possibility is the potential catastrophic event of a reduction of strangulated, unhealthy piece of bowel within the abdominal cavity. The gangrenous bowel may very quickly break open and spill intestinal contents into the abdomen.

At the first sign of strangulation, all attempts at reduction should cease and the patient should be operated upon immediately.

Where Is Elective Hernia Surgery Performed?

Hernia correction by surgery is performed in an outpatient facility for approximately 90% of patients.

MediCare has accepted the financial responsibility for the care of eligible patients who need hernia surgery, but has mandated that the repair be performed without hospitalization whenever possible. Third-party payors, such as insurance companies, have followed the lead of Medicare and pay for hospitalization only in unusual circumstances. In California, all Medicare patients are reviewed pre-operatively by the California Medical Review Institute (CMRI). CMRI nearly always refuses admission to the hospital for inguinal hernia surgery. Unusual recurrent hernias, bilateral hernias, or patients with severe medical problems (such as a 40% reduction in heart output), are *considered* for hospitalization. CMRI and private insurance companies usually stipulate hospitalization can be obtained post-operatively, if a problem develops during the operation or in the post-operative period. Difficulties must be carefully documented in the hospital record and the documentation is reviewed by CMRI or the insurance company before payment for your stay is authorized.

Thus the use of outpatient facilities has become routine for hernia surgeries over the past five years. If a transfer to a hospital is necessary, this is easily accomplished.

For those who wish greater detail, the following is provided.

Typical Inguinal Hernia Surgical Technique

The patient is placed on the operating table, on his or her back, with feet and head level. If the hernia is large, or involves intestine, the head may be lowered approximately 15 degrees, to ease the return of the contents from the hernia into the abdominal cavity. The patient's arms are usually comfortably extended onto padded arm boards at about 45 degrees from the body. Anesthetic techniques are discussed in greater detail in Chapter Thirteen. The patient must not have had anything to eat or drink for at least six hours before arrival at the operating room. An "IV" (intravenous catheter) is placed in a vein in the patient's hand or forearm. This is used pre-operatively to allow the introduction of intravenous antibiotics. (The use of pre-operative antibiotics has been shown to reduce the incidence of infection.) The IV line allows easy introduction of anesthetic agents and fluids into the circulation to compensate for the pre-operative dehydration. The lower abdomen and groin area is shaved. Removal of body hair makes the incision and suturing easier and the bandage can be removed later without pulling hairs. Some patients prefer to shave themselves, but this is not recommended. The groin and surrounding area is carefully washed with a soap, followed by a prep solution, usually one containing iodine, such as Betadine®. If the patient is allergic to iodine, other products, such as Hibiclens® and Phisohex® are substituted. These products are used to "sterilize" the skin and can be somewhat irritating. During the application, the nurses are very careful to prevent pooling or accumulation of these solutions. (However, in spite of these efforts, post-operative irritation of the skin does occasionally occur.) Surgical drapes are then applied. These are sterile, usually paper, and have adherent surfaces so that they stick to the patient's skin. They are placed in a manner so as to expose a rectangular area of skin slightly larger than the area of intended skin incision. Considerable effort is made to avoid placing these drapes over the patient's hair-bearing areas. Lastly, a large, sterile drape with a small window is placed over the area and is draped over the entire patient from neck to toe. This creates a surgically sterile field for the surgeon and the operating team. A divider is placed between the patient's head and the operative area, so that the patient may converse, cough or sneeze, without contaminating the operative area.

> **For those who wish *even greater* detail in the description, the following is provided.**

A Description of Surgery

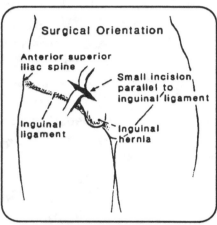

Figure 4-G

1. A small incision is made near the skin crease at the junction of abdomen and thigh. Gentle pressure is applied by surgeon and assistant with one of their hands while the incision is made and bleeding is minimized. Actually, there typically is very little bleeding during the procedure.

2. Small retractors are now introduced and these hold the subcutaneous tissue away from the center of the operative field. The external ring is then identified and a small incision is made in the external oblique aponeurosis. The fibers of the external oblique aponeurosis are lifted from

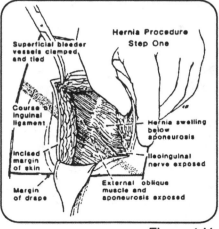

Figure 4-H

the underlying structures and the incision is extended into the external ring, exposing the cord structures and the entire inguinal canal. The ileoinguinal nerve lies just deep to this aponeurosis, and is carefully spared.

3. The edges of the divided external oblique aponeurosis are then grasped, one at a time, and the underlying tissue is gently dissected from it, to expose the internal oblique muscle medially and the Poupart ligament laterally.

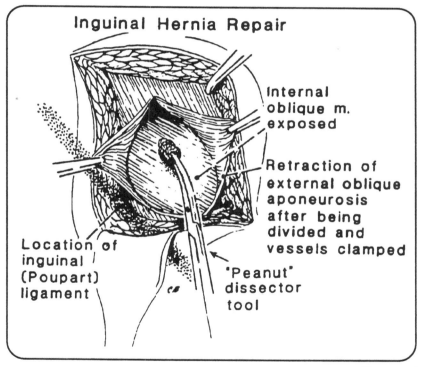

Figure 4-I

4. The hernia sac is then identified by dissecting in this recently exposed tissue layer. If the patient is awake, he or she is asked to cough or strain and to demonstrate the hernia. See figure 4-J, which shows a direct hernia, separate from the cord structures.

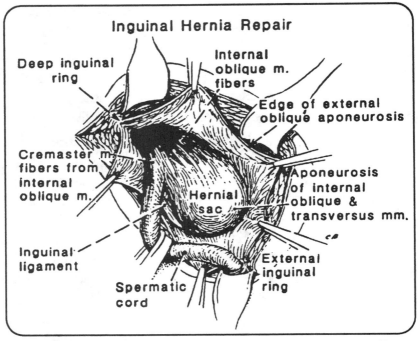

Inguinal Hernia Repair

Deep inguinal
ring

Internal
oblique m.
fibers

Edge of external
oblique aponeurosis

Cremaster m.
fibers from
internal
oblique m.

Hernial
sac

Aponeurosis
of internal
oblique &
transversus mm.

Inguinal
ligament

Spermatic
cord

External
inguinal
ring

Figure 4-J

5. The hernia sac is then dissected from the surrounding tissue to its point of origin. If the hernia is indirect, the dissection proceeds to the internal inguinal ring. This dissection is very gentle and specific. Usually, the surgeon uses a moistened gauze placed over his finger, or a "peanut", to "wipe" the tissues and thereby separate them one from the other. The sac is then treated. If the sac is shaped like a sausage, and is easily dissected from the surrounding tissue, its contents are returned into the abdomen and the sac is tied at its origin, or invaginated. At this stage, the inguinal floor is examined for further defects, the cord structures and vessels leading to the testicles are identified and spared, and any extra tissue such as fat (a lipoma of the cord) is identified and removed. See figure 4-K.

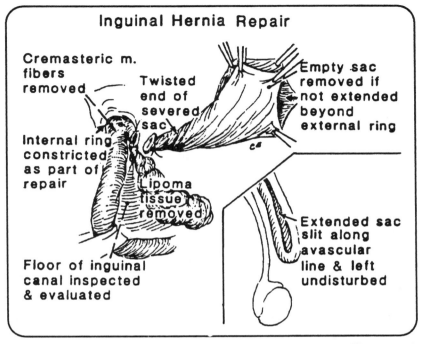

Inguinal Hernia Repair

Cremasteric m. fibers removed

Twisted end of severed sac

Empty sac removed if not extended beyond external ring

Internal ring constricted as part of repair

Lipoma tissue removed

Floor of inguinal canal inspected & evaluated

Extended sac slit along avascular line & left undisturbed

Figure 4-K

6. Cremasteric muscle fibers, which are a continuation of the internal oblique muscle, proceeding along with the cord structures, are now carefully identified and partially divided. This division also makes the total diameter of the cord structures relatively small, and facilitates creation of a small internal ring, which is so important to a successful repair.

7. The distal sac, if it does not extend beyond the inguinal canal, is removed. If the sac extends beyond the canal, dissection is limited to avoid injury to the blood supply to the testicle. Instead, the sac is simply opened along an avascular line to hopefully prevent later development of a hydrocele. Dr. George Wantz has written extensively on this dissection and has shown, in his practice, that attempts to remove the sac in its entirety may cause injury to the veins to the testicle.

8. The floor of the inguinal canal is inspected and its strength or weakness evaluated. Women in general, or young and muscular males frequently do not need further exploration or repair.

9. The posterior floor of the inguinal canal is now repaired, according to the presentation and the need of that area. With knife, and then scissors, the transversalis aponeurosis is opened throughout the length of the floor of the canal. (See figure 4-L) The fat between this fascia and the peritoneum (preperitoneal fat) is dissected to expose the lateral and medial margins of the inguinal floor. About 10 percent of patients have a very, very weak and wide inguinal canal floor. With these patients, a piece of strengthening mesh is inserted and sutured in place posterior to (behind) the wide floor before the closure is started.

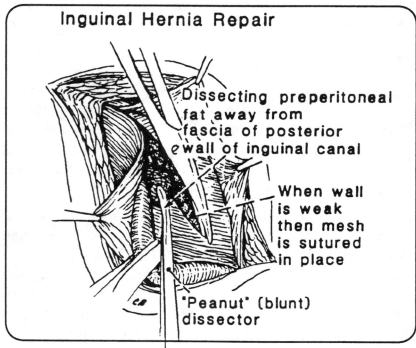

Inguinal Hernia Repair

Dissecting preperitoneal fat away from fascia of posterior wall of inguinal canal

When wall is weak then mesh is sutured in place

"Peanut" (blunt) dissector

Figure 4-L

10. Closure is performed in a "vest-over-pants" manner, using a running suture to secure the Iliopubic fascia to the underlying surface of the transversalis, then a second layer closing the transversalis fascia to the Poupart's ligament. A knot is placed *away from* the pubic bone, for pressure on this knot, if placed near the pubic bone, causes pain later during sexual activity.

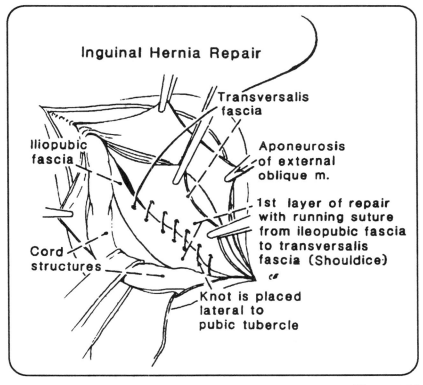

Inguinal Hernia Repair

Transversalis fascia

Iliopubic fascia

Aponeurosis of external oblique m.

1st layer of repair with running suture from ileopubic fascia to transversalis fascia (Shouldice)

Cord structures

Knot is placed lateral to pubic tubercle

Figure 4-M

11. During this two-layer closure, the internal ring is closed very snugly about the cord structures. The genitofemoral nerve, with some of the associated cremasteric fibers, may be sacrificed, or brought out separately, through a notch in the closure.

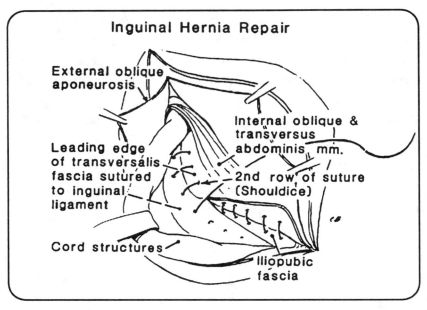

Figure 4-N

12. After the repair is completed, the patient is asked to strain or cough again, at which time the integrity of the repair is checked.

During this entire procedure, the assistant and the scrub nurse are working actively to provide the best operative care possible. The operation proceeds quickly. The hands of the nurse, assistant, and surgeon are all continually working as a team. To a surgeon, this is a joy to behold.

---

13. In some patients, the surgeon may elect to reinforce the repair. Then, a piece of mesh or Gore-tex® is selected and cut to fit the area and is inserted into place to supplement the existing repair. This is held in place with tiny, extremely strong sutures.

14. A "keyhole" is produced in the patch to allow passage of the cord structures. The ends of the patch, superior and lateral to this keyhole, are allowed to remain in place and support the superior and lateral aspects of the area.

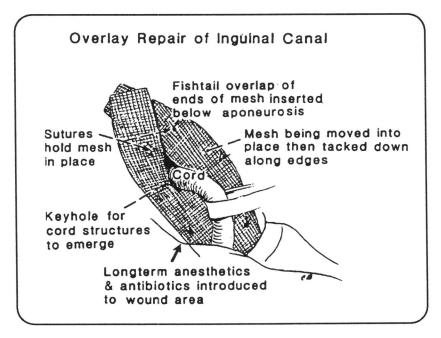

Overlay Repair of Inguinal Canal

Fishtail overlap of ends of mesh inserted below aponeurosis

Sutures hold mesh in place

Mesh being moved into place then tacked down along edges

Cord

Keyhole for cord structures to emerge

Longterm anesthetics & antibiotics introduced to wound area

Figure 4-O

15. At the commencement of the closure, the operative field and mesh may be washed repeatedly with solution of antibiotics. This step is omitted if pre-operative intravenous antibiotics are given. The use of antibiotics, either intravenously or intra-operatively, prevents post-operative wound infection and has a low incidence of side effects.

16. During closure, the area is infiltrated with a long-acting anesthetic to relieve pain for the first six to eight hours immediately after surgery.

17. The divided edges of the external oblique aponeurosis are then sutured to one another over the cord structures, recreating an external ring. Once again, the ilioinguinal nerve is carefully spared. See figure 4-P.

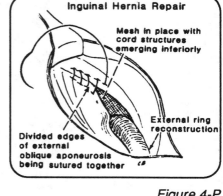

Inguinal Hernia Repair

Mesh in place with cord structures emerging inferiorly

External ring reconstruction

Divided edges of external oblique aponeurosis being sutured together

Figure 4-P

18. The subcutaneous tissue, and its fascia, may be closed with a running absorbable suture.

Skin Closure

Concealed suture in subcuticular layer of skin

Central point exposed loop to be cut upon removal

Both ends of continuous suture tied together for later removal

Figure 4-Q

19. The incision is then closed using a delicate suture which leaves very few skin marks and a fine scar. Other techniques may include the use of sterile strips of adhesive, simple skin sutures, or clips.

20. A dry sterile gauze dressing is applied and taped in place.

21. If the operation has been performed using local anesthesia, it takes about an hour. The patient is able to move him or herself from the operating table onto the gurney for transport from the operating room to recovery room. The patient usually stays in the recovery room for about 45 minutes, until he or she has taken fluids, walked, and emptied the bladder.

22. If the patient has been given a general anesthetic, the operation takes about 30 to 45 minutes. The difference

in the length of time between the two procedures is related to the use of the local anesthetic and the greater wait for it to become effective. On completion of the surgery, when using general anesthetic, the patient is gently lifted from the operating table onto the gurney and transported to the recovery room by the anesthesiologist and the nurse. In the recovery room, the patient is allowed to awaken. Later, fluids are offered and the patient is assisted to ambulate and empty his or her bladder. This recovery time takes about one to one-and-a-half hours.

Are There Any Other Methods of Hernia Repair?

The Cooper ligament, or "McVay", form of hernia repair, when properly performed, is an excellent operation. This technique has been popular for many years and is still used by many surgeons today.

The Shouldice, or Canadian repair has been used with great success . It was popularized by the Shouldice clinic in Toronto Canada, but is actually similar to the original Bassini repair. Surgeons throughout the world and in the United States are using this technique with increasing frequency.

The Marcy repair is sometimes used on young and muscular individuals.

Of course, other methods of repair exist, and are used, according to the preference of the surgeon.

A McVay or Cooper Ligament Repair

A study of patients receiving the Cooper ligament repair was discussed and updated by Jacques Barbier, et. al., of France. The series, which included histories of patients operated on between 1970 and 1978, reported excellent results.

About 70% of the cases in the study were followed for an average period of 12.19 years. (Most studies follow the patient for approximately one year.) The recurrence rate of 4% for the primary hernia repair was an excellent result, and actually would have reflected a rate of less than 2%, based on a typical *one* year follow-up.

After dissecting the floor of the inguinal canal, as in the other repairs, an incision is made in the floor of the inguinal canal. The Cooper ligament and the surrounding structures are exposed. The femoral sheath and the external iliac vessels are retracted laterally.

The hernial protrusion is then reduced, and interrupted sutures (possibly 2-0 silk or neurolon) are placed. (See figure 4-R) After all of the sutures are in place, the amount of tension that will be created by tying them is evaluated, and a relaxing incision is made in the anterior

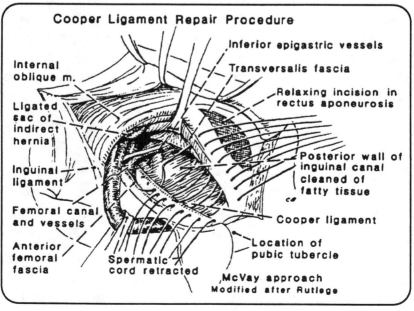

Figure 4-R

rectus sheath, if needed. The sutures are then tied. These sutures approximate the musculofascial segment of the transversus muscle, medially, to the Cooper ligament, the pectineus fascia, the anterior femoral sheath, and the reflection of the inguinal ligament, laterally.

The Shouldice Repair

Dr. George Wantz of the New York Hospital/Cornell Medical Center has been using a procedure called "Canadian hernioplasty", or "Shouldice Repair", since 1970.

Dr. Wantz discussed the Shouldice technique and reviewed his experiences in *The World Journal of Surgery* in 1989. Dr. Wantz reported on a series of 4,622 inguinal hernia repairs using the Shouldice technique with a 1 to 20 year follow-up and a 1.3% recurrence rate.

He discussed the Canadian hernia repair as follows: *"The structures are approximated in a more refined and precise manner and, rather than abutting the layers at the edge with one layer of interrupted sutures, the various layers are imbricated [overlapped] with continuous sutures. The repair begins with a suture merely anchored in the ileopubic tract near the pubic cubicle. The edge of the lateral aponeuroticofascial segment is sutured to the undersurface of the medial segment. Next, the edge of the transverse aponeurotic arch, with its attached muscle, is sutured to the shelving edge of the inguinal ligament. The current suture of choice for this layer of imbrication is polypropylene.*

"The double seam advantageously avoids gaps and neutralizes errors in judgment of the integrity of the aponeuroticofascial layers. Also, suture holes in the femoral sheath and the transverse aponeurosis, which could be potential sites of recurrent herniations, are covered. Continuous suture, which must not be pulled tight, distributes tension evenly. There is remarkably little tension on the

suture line and relaxing incisions are customarily not made. The absence of suture line tension undoubtedly contributes to the good results and the benign convalescence.

"The proximal stump of the cremaster muscle is used in repair of the deep [inguinal] ring. This stump is incorporated with the sutures in the femoral sheath and sewed to the undersurface of the transverse aponeurotic arch. It, therefore, nearly encircles the spermatic cord and obliterates

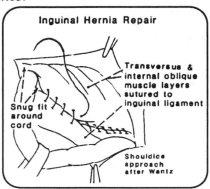

Figure 4-S

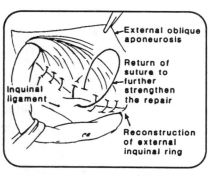

Figure 4-T

the deep ring to touch, but does not squeeze the cord as much as prevent the cord from sliding back and forth within the ring.

"This reconstruction of the deep ring is much tighter than that performed by many surgeons. Constriction of the cord at the deep ring does not cause ischemic orchitis [problems with the blood supply to the testicle]." Reprinted with the permission of Dr. George Wantz, and Société Internationale.

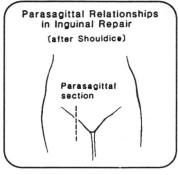

Figure 4-U

To illustrate, refer to figures 4-M and 4-N, earlier in this Chapter. Two more layers of repair follow, shown in figures 4-S and 4-T.

To further illustrate this, Dr. Bridgman has chosen a parasagittal view, as demonstrated in

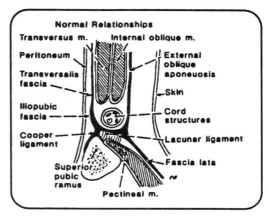

Figure 4-V

figure 4-U. The normal anatomy is shown in figure 4-V, and the completed Shouldice repair, in figure 4-W.

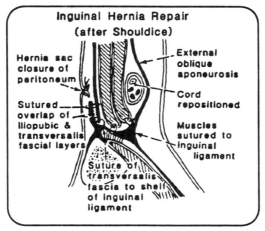

Figure 4-W

The Marcy Repair

The Marcy repair has not been illustrated. It consists of the repair of the internal ring area, after treatment of the sac. This repair is used when the patient's inguinal canal has a strong floor, but a dilated internal ring.

Inguinal Hernias In Females

Indirect inguinal hernias along the inguinal canal do occur in females. Female patients with an inguinal hernia *occasionally* complain of pain in the lower abdomen yet do not show a bulge at the external inguinal ring area. The physician should consider an inguinal hernia when examining women for lower abdominal pain. Such patients must be examined carefully, in the standing position, while straining, in order to demonstrate the hernia. Even then, the hernia may not protrude outside of the inguinal canal.

In females, the hernia sac may adhere to the round ligament (there is no spermatic cord). The sac may contain the fallopian tube or ovary (particularly in younger patients). The round ligament does not serve any useful function and may be removed from the canal at the time of the removal of the sac. Therefore, the entire internal ring area may be tightly closed. With these exceptions, the female anatomy (muscles, fascia,

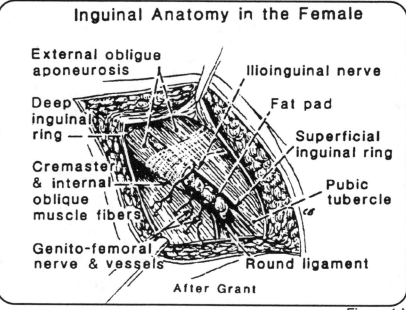

Inguinal Anatomy in the Female

External oblique aponeurosis

Ilioinguinal nerve

Deep inguinal ring —

Fat pad

Superficial inguinal ring

Cremaster & internal oblique muscle fibers

Pubic tubercle

Genito-femoral nerve & vessels

Round ligament

After Grant

Figure 4-X

and nerves) is similar to that of males. A *recurrent* inguinal hernia is rare in women.

Women have a tendency to develop a femoral hernia after repair of an inguinal hernia, particularly if the repair is performed with tension in the suture line. Therefore, whenever an inguinal hernia is being repaired in a female patient, the technical alternatives available include:

1) Closure of the femoral canal and simple closure of the femoral ring at the time of the inguinal hernia repair; and

2) A tension-free repair of the inguinal hernia to prevent distortion of the femoral canal.

"Sliding" Inguinal Hernias

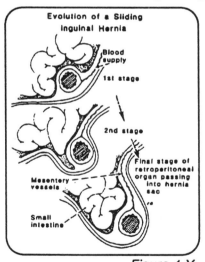

Figure 4-Y

Occasionally, the hernia sac is quite large and the wall of the sac, as it extends into the hernia, carries with it the wall of the adjacent organ, such as a loop of intestine. This is a "sliding hernia". The illustration, figure 4-Y, shows the development of a slider, with the sac wall including a piece of the colon.

Large inguinal hernias on the left commonly have the wall of the sigmoid colon as part of the sac wall. The large intestine, even the appendix, may be involved as part of the sac wall on the right side. The bladder wall occasionally joins the sac of large direct inguinal hernias on either side. In the female, especially infants and children, a sliding hernia may contain portions of the female reproductive tract, such as a fallopian tube or an ovary. Naturally, great care must be exercised in the treatment of these sliding hernia sacs, for simple high ligation of the hernia sac could not be performed without injuring the organ. The involved organ must first be recognized, and reduced without injury. The blood supply to the organ must always be carefully preserved.

Summary

If you have a hernia, chances are it is an inguinal hernia. They are the most frequent occurring type of hernia and, fortunately, are usually easy to diagnose and easy to treat.

Inguinal hernias may be indirect (congenital) or direct (acquired) and different factors contribute to the development of each.

Early, accurate diagnosis of an inguinal hernia is important. Many patients "discover" the hernia themselves when they notice a lump or bulge in the groin area.

Advances in modern medicine have made inguinal hernias much easier to treat than in years past. Today, the preferred method of surgical repair usually can be scheduled to the convenience of the patient — and requires far less interruption of their daily routine.

There are several fine surgical methods of inguinal hernia repair that have been developed. For those "scientifically-inclined" readers who would like to learn about these methods in greater detail, descriptions are provided in the preceding text.

Most inguinal hernia surgery patients experience minimal discomfort and return to their near-normal activities within three to four days post-operatively. Convalescence usually takes about three weeks, during which time *truly heavy* lifting should be avoided.

Chapter Five

Recurrent Inguinal Hernias

The trust that patients place in their physicians is hard-earned; today's medical professionals must know more than ever before *and* are required by law to spend great effort to frequently update their knowledge and skills in post-graduate studies.

Despite the qualifications and competence of physicians and surgeons, the complexity (and, indeed unpredictability) of the human body results in a small percentage of "partially" successful treatments, i.e., procedures that are initially successful, but which ultimately require further or secondary treatment.

In the case of inguinal hernias, the incidence of recurrence (or having to repair them again) is relatively low, yet must be acknowledged.

Approximately 550,000 inguinal hernias are operated on each *year* in the United States alone. Approximately 100,000 of these are performed on *recurrent* inguinal hernias. Interestingly, this apparent overall recurrence rate of up to 18 percent varies greatly from practice to practice.

Problems of Recurrence

Several problems, some minor and some major, may result from recurrence of an inguinal hernia. Not only is the patient subject to a second surgery, but he or she is again exposed to the risks which accompany any surgical procedure. Furthermore, performing the operation through scar tissue of the previous operation may cause increased problems in the operative site. Neuralgia (or wound pain), numbness in the groin, and an increased possibility of injury to the testicle, are just a few of the problems that have been reported after re-dissection and repair of recurrent inguinal hernias. Moreover, repair of recurrent inguinal hernias is followed by an increased incidence of recurrences, when compared to initial repairs. For these reasons, it is very important to make every effort at the initial operation to avoid a recurrence.

Incidence of Recurrent Hernias

Surgical literature is replete with articles which discuss the problem of recurrence in inguinal hernias, and suggest alternative approaches and techniques for correction.

The British Journal Of Surgery (1988) contains an excellent personal series reported by Dr. A. J. Marsden with 287 recurrent inguinal hernias repaired using four different techniques. The overall recurrence rate (27 failures in 287 operations) of nine percent, was disappointing to the author.

In the Netherland's Journal Of Surgery (1989), Van Ooijen reported a total of 96 recurrent inguinal hernias repaired between 1978 and 1983. They followed their patients for an average of 5.2 years and detected a recurrence rate of nine percent in those patients who were available for follow-up. Unfortunately, 19 percent of the patients could not be located for follow-up examination. The doctors used Teflon mesh to repair 58 of the recurrent inguinal hernias and were favorably impressed with the advantages offered by the insertion of this prosthetic mesh.

In *Hernia*, Nyhus and Condon tabulate recurrence rates of inguinal hernias from previously published series. Their list revealed a recurrence rate from one to ten percent. Recurrence rates for *recurrent* inguinal hernia repair were estimated at five to 35 percent.

On the other hand,Lichtenstein, Shulman, and Amid have written multiple articles in the surgical literature in the past two years, and have cited a recurrence rate of 0.25 percent to 1.6 percent with a follow-up of 91 percent of their patients.

In summary, inguinal hernias do recur after repair with some frequency; and, second repairs are subject to an even greater incidence of recurrence. Surgeons are working very hard to eliminate this problem.

The wide variation in the recurrence rates probably seems unusual to the lay person. The patient "selection", however, can account for much of this. Patients may be quite varied. They may have hernias that are extremely large and extremely difficult to care for. Age, or other health factors, may contribute to recurrences or repair failures. Some surgeons specialize in surgery in young children, others in the elderly. Some surgeons limit their practice to elective surgery, while others see many patients in emergency situations. These varying patient populations will significantly alter the success rate of the surgeon's hernia operations.

One other variable that is extremely important in reviewing these statistics is the follow-up rate. The follow-up rate, varying from 80 to 90 percent, means that 10 to 20 percent of the patients have not been available to provide follow-up information about their condition.

When a series reports a recurrent rate of one percent, but a follow-up rate of 80 percent (where 20 percent of the patients could not be located), it doesn't seem prudent to assume that there has been simply a one percent recurrence rate. It would seem more reasonable to suggest that the recurrence rate is between one and 21 percent.

Causes of Recurrence

What are the possible causes of all of these recurrences? **Recurrences occur when there is some deviation from the normal formula of tension-free rejoining of good tissue to good tissue.** A most obvious reason for failure is the patient's tissue itself. Some patients simply do not have good muscle or connective tissue. Some patients do not exercise enough, do not eat sufficient protein or may drink too much alcohol. It is obvious to the operating surgeon that the muscles and fascia of such a patient are not strong and therefore, suturing them together may not produce a solid wall of supporting tissue. Dr. Erle Peacock has shown that there can be a degenerative process within the connective tissue in some individuals, possibly related to the aging process. There are several medical conditions which involve congenital weakness of the connective tissue. Such degenerative processes in the connective tissue may be important factors in patients who develop a recurrence later than one year from the surgical procedure.

Many patients tend to put unusual and repeated pressure on their wound. Some people are chronically constipated and may think it perfectly normal to strain vigorously with every bowel movement. Over time, such straining applies unusual pressure on the wound area and may result in an eventual wound breakdown. Similarly, some men may have a prostate condition which results in a gradual closing of the urinary outlet. This straining to urinate, once again causes continued pressure or straining against the abdominal wall, and may contribute to eventual breakdown of the hernia. Women, in particular, may develop a stricture of their bladder outlet, causing them to strain while attempting to urinate.

Many people do not maintain a reasonable exercise program. Some simply do not exercise at all. Others exercise, but do not stimulate the muscles of the abdominal trunk. Exercises, such as sit-ups and simultaneous twisting, are important in maintaining the tone of the abdominal muscles and fascia. Even those persons in good overall condition should twist, do sit-ups, and perform exercises which will strengthen their abdominal muscles. See exercises, illustrated in Chapter Two.

About Weight

Obesity is considered by many to be an important contributing factor to recurrences. Some surgeons refuse to operate on patients who are 15 percent over their ideal body weight. These surgeons simply ask patients to go home, go on a diet, and return after satisfactory weight reduction. This is a very reasonable approach to the problem of fatty infiltration into the area. Fat does infiltrate the muscles and fascia; fat also adds to the volume in the area and distorts the tissue out of normal alignment. Attempts to attach fat cells to fat cells during surgery does not produce a solid repair.

Other Contributing Factors

One significant problem may occur immediately post-operatively, after administration of a general anesthesia. The patient may strain vigorously as he or she awakens and break open their repair. This is one reason why some surgeons try to avoid general anesthesia.

Incisions may become infected. When this happens the sutures may become infected as well, with subsequent wound breakdown. Multifilamented sutures, such as silk or cotton, are particularly prone to develop infections. The bacteria may survive for years within the spaces of the woven or braided fibers of these sutures. Then, often years later, the bacteria will multiply and form an abscess.

Unusual bleeding may occur during a repair. The usual hernia repair is quite free of bleeding. Most vessels are seen before they are cut and the ends are sealed by ligature or cautery. However, during the suturing of multiple layers required for closure, the surgeon uses needles which penetrate the tissue. Every effort is made to avoid piercing a blood vessel, but this is not always possible. The needle penetrates out of sight during its passage through the tissue and occasional bleeding after suturing does occur. There is then a pooling of blood in the wound which distorts the tissue and once again may contribute to a recurrence.

Some patients, such as those with *asthma or emphysema,* have extreme respiratory problems and often are literally straining for every breath. They not only have difficulty exhaling and are constantly putting pressure on their abdomen in order to breathe, they frequently have an associated cough. These patients suffer a particularly high incidence of recurrence.

Any discussion of the causes of recurrences would be incomplete without inclusion of the significant problem caused by *smoking*. Patients who smoke often have chronic bronchitis and produce extra secretions. The mechanism for removal of these secretions is damaged by the smoking or bronchitis. The lungs are unable to sweep the secretions and debris out of the lungs in a normal manner and, therefore, the patient must "lift" the secretions by coughing. Every post-operative patient will tell you it is painful to cough. Smokers probably cough 200 to 300 times daily. A non-smoker may not cough at all. Repeated coughing is irritating to the wound and is undoubtedly a contributing factor to recurrences. Some surgeons actually refuse to repair recurrent inguinal hernias for any patients who continue to smoke. Others make a real effort to help the patient stop smoking for a brief period, pre-operatively. If the patient can stop smoking for one to two months before surgery, the post-operative course may be significantly easier for the patient.

Individual variations in anatomy of the area are important when discussing recurrences. Individuals' muscles and fascia do vary. Some patients have a wide separation between the muscles in this area. This and other anatomical differences or variations, from one patient to another, are obvious to the anatomist or surgeon and effect the surgical outcome.

Finally, and of equal importance to all of the foregoing, the surgeon and his experience seem to be demonstrably significant in the prevention of recurrences. More and more experts express the opinion that experienced hernia surgeons, who are dedicated to the task, have a significantly reduced rate of recurrence. This opinion was well expressed in an editorial in the American Journal of Surgery in September, 1990, by Maximo Deysine, M.D. and Harry S. Soroff, M.D., of the Department of Surgery, University Hospital, at State University of New York at Stonybrook, New York. They stated:

"*The results of surgery for a primary inguinal hernia are determined by the incidence of recurrence, a complication that indicates the need for re-operation. Repairs of inguinal hernia are generally carried out by two categories of surgeons: those who perform herniorrhaphies* [hernia repair] *occasionally, as part of a broad-based general surgical practice; and those who have developed a special interest in hernias and operate on them exclusive of other procedures. In the United States, the results obtained by these two groups of surgeons, as published in current literature, appear to be significantly different. While national figures reveal a recurrence rate of 10% for primary and 25% for recurrent inguinal hernia, the herniorrhaphists* [surgeons who specialize in surgical hernia repair] *report recurrence rates of only 1% for primary and 5% for recurrent inguinal hernias. The magnitude of the difference between these two groups can best be appreciated by comparing figures based on the current number of hernia repairs. Of the approximately 550,000 inguinal herniorrhaphies performed annually in this country, the 10% and 15% recurrence rate would result in some 55,000 recurrences after the first procedure and 13,750 after the second and 3,437 after the third. In sharp contrast, if those original 550,000 herniorrhaphies had been performed by surgeons dedicated to that field, at the reported 1% and 5% recurrence rate, only 13 patients would need a fourth operation.*

"*The hernia service created in 1980 demonstrates the merits of standardization. The service is directed by a senior faculty member who originally planned the care of the patient population by programming a detailed, pre-operative, operative, and post-operative protocol suited for the progressive training of surgical residents. The protocol is divided into 80 different steps to be sequentially implemented in the management of each patient. To date, the service* *has directed operations on 1,754 patients, with a 75% seven-year follow-up; a recurrence rate of 2%; an infection rate of 0.3%, and one death. Moreover the recurrence and infection rates of this program were found to be significantly better (p<0.005) than those achieved at the same institution by board-certified general surgeons who had previously performed herniorrhaphies as part of a larger and varied general surgical practice, assisting the same group of residents. In addition, such reorganization led to significantly better results than those previously reported in current literature for patients over 65 years of age. Furthermore, early operation on patients of all ages considered by strict criteria to be at high risk produced an 85% reduction in the incidence of emergency surgery for incarceration and strangulation. As an added benefit to our institution, this reorganization permitted an improved follow-up."* Reprinted with the permission of Maximo Deysine and *The American Journal of Surgery*.

What Are the Hazards of Repair in a Recurrent Inguinal Hernia?

A recurrent inguinal hernia is often more difficult to repair, because the surgery must be performed through considerable scar tissue. **This scar tissue frequently obscures the usual "landmarks" available to the surgeon and makes exposure of the vessels and nerves in this area more difficult.**

Patients with repeated inguinal hernia repairs frequently have numbness in the groin after surgery. Less common, but more annoying, is the persistence of pain in the area. This is called neuralgia.

Lastly, any repair in a male patient must leave room for the vessels and the cord structures which supply the testicle. **Unusual pressure on these vessels may decrease the circulation to the testicle and result in atrophy of it.** Atrophy means that the testicle is reduced in size and may therefore be less functional. A. J. Marsden reported three cases of testicular atrophy in a series of 287 operations for recurrent inguinal hernias. Although statistically a "small" problem, it is a significant one to each patient who suffers this complication.

What are the Methods Currently Used to Repair a Recurrent Inguinal Hernia?

Dr. Lloyd Nyhus and George Wantz make an incision superior to (above) the inguinal canal, dissect through the abdominal wall, to approach the inguinal hernia posteriorly (from behind). They favor the posterior approach, and feel that the improved results warrant the additional dissection. There is excellent exposure of both inguinal and femoral areas in this approach. One particular advantage of this approach is the insertion of a

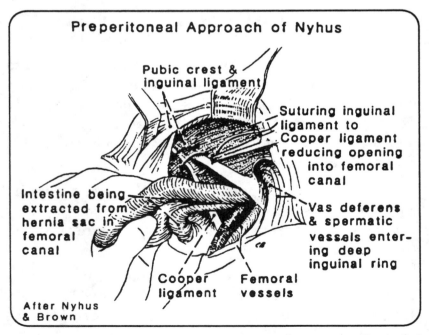

Preperitoneal Approach of Nyhus

Pubic crest & inguinal ligament

Suturing inguinal ligament to Cooper ligament reducing opening into femoral canal

Intestine being extracted from hernia sac in femoral canal

Vas deferens & spermatic vessels entering deep inguinal ring

Cooper ligament

Femoral vessels

After Nyhus & Brown

Figure 5-A

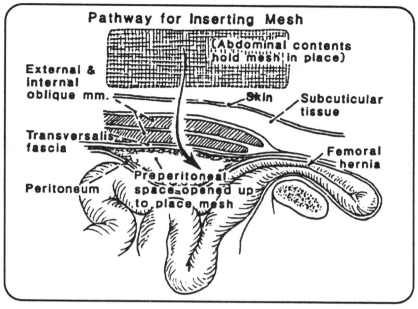

Figure 5-B

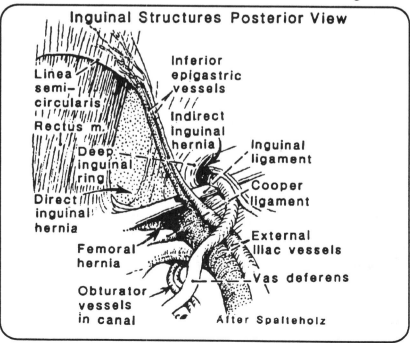

Figure 5-C

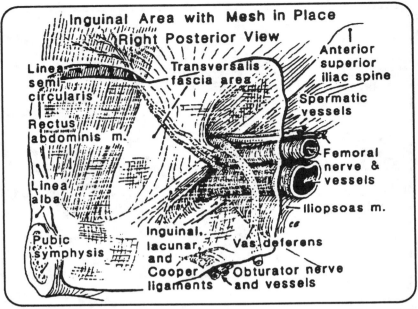

Inguinal Area with Mesh in Place
Right Posterior View

Linea semi circularis

Transversalis fascia area

Anterior superior iliac spine

Spermatic vessels

Rectus abdominis m.

Femoral nerve & vessels

Linea alba

Iliopsoas m.

Pubic symphysis

Inguinal, lacunar, and Cooper ligaments

Vas deferens

Obturator nerve and vessels

Figure 5-D

mesh or patch between the abdominal wall and the abdominal contents. Then, the normal pressure from the peritoneum (which encloses the abdominal contents) serves to hold the mesh in place.

Dr. Rene Stoppa describes a somewhat different approach in which a large piece of mesh is inserted, once again from the posterior aspect of the abdominal wall. Dr. Stoppa uses a midline incision which offers the advantage of exposure of both inguinal areas simultaneously. After exposing the inguinal areas, and repairing the hernias, Dr. Stoppa then inserts a large piece of mesh covering the entire anterior abdominal wall and a considerable portion of the lateral abdominal wall, as well. Dr. Stoppa reviewed 230 cases of voluminous (or very large) groin hernias, in The World Journal of Surgery, in 1989, and found a recurrence rate of only 3.4 percent. These are excellent results, in patients with such large and difficult problems.

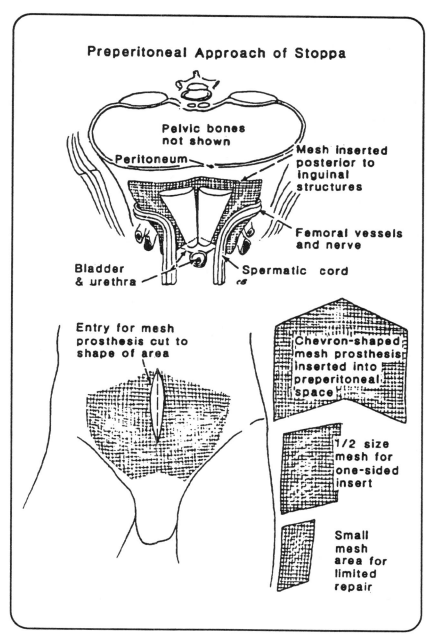

Preperitoneal Approach of Stoppa

Pelvic bones
not shown

Peritoneum

Mesh inserted
posterior to
inguinal
structures

Femoral vessels
and nerve

Bladder
& urethra

Spermatic cord

Entry for mesh
prosthesis cut to
shape of area

Chevron-shaped
mesh prosthesis
inserted into
preperitoneal
space

1/2 size
mesh for
one-sided
insert

Small
mesh
area for
limited
repair

Figure 5-E

Another most innovative and exciting technique is the use of polypropylene mesh rolled into the form of a plug and inserted into the defect and sutured in place. Recently discussed by Drs. Shulman, Amid and Lichtenstein in *The Archives of Surgery* in February, 1990, 1,402 operations are described in which the plug was used on virtually all patients. 91 percent of the cases was available for follow-up and the recurrence rate was a low 1.6 percent. They preferred not to expose the entire area of the previous repair, but simply located the defect and inserted the plug into it. A one-inch wide strip of polypropylene mesh was rolled until the diameter of the roll (plug) equaled that of the defect. In discussing this technique, Dr. Shulman stresses the importance that the plug be large enough so that its insertion creates a "snug fit". The defect is then simply sutured so that the plug is held in place. This results in a tension-free repair. The procedure is performed under a local or epidural anesthetic, with the patient awake, able to cough or strain, and demonstrate the hernia. After the repair, the patient is asked to once again cough or strain and demonstrate its repair. The authors also cite the added benefit of a more pleasant postoperative course, because of the limited dissection and the absence of tension in the repair. The use of a plug is illustrated in Chapter Six, Femoral Hernias.

A different approach to the same problem consists of dissection through the old scar, with insertion of a piece of polypropylene mesh into the floor of the inguinal canal. The mesh is placed posterior, or deep, to the floor of the inguinal canal. Dr. Bendavid utilized this technique as on 28 patients in the Shouldice Hospital in Ontario, Canada. He experienced very few complications, and only one recurrence.

Another distinguished surgeon, Dr. Arthur Gilbert, also approaches the inguinal canal directly and, if the posterior floor is weak, inserts a piece of polypropylene mesh deep to that floor. Dr. Gilbert reported 2,325 inguinal and femoral hernia repairs in 1987. His series was not for recurrent inguinal hernias alone, but the series is valuable to mention, as it includes a technique using the approach through the inguinal canal. allowing insertion of mesh deep to the canal. He cited the advantages of outpatient treatment in 91 percent of his cases and early return to work. 95 percent of his patients return to their usual work or activity by the end of the first week. He stated that exceptions to this early return were usually *"patients funded by workers compensation"* and *"patients doing strenuous work requiring use, primarily, of their sinew"*.

Dr. Stanley Berliner uses a similar technique, and inserts a patch of Gore-tex®.

The foregoing discussion suggests the many alternatives available to the surgeon and to the patient, at the time of surgical repair of a recurrent inguinal hernia. Patients vary greatly in the size of their defects, and the apparent strength of their tissues, as well as other factors, and, therefore, each patient might be considered individually and the surgery tailored to fit their problem. The Stoppa approach seems an obvious choice for large and bilateral hernias. The Nyhus approach is extremely effective in difficult recurrent hernias on one side. The anterior approach is valuable for small defects, allowing the surgeon to expose the area, and then make a decision at the time of surgery whether to insert a plug, or a sheet of mesh or Gore-tex®, or even to utilize the patient's own strong tissues. Making a decision at the time of surgery, based on the "situation and terrain" has many advantages.

Summary

It is a fact of life that a certain number of patients will have a recurrence of their hernias following an otherwise successful and uneventful repair. All of the reasons for recurrence are not known, however, age, tissue condition, lack of proper exercise, excess weight, smoking, and unusual pressure on the area of the initial hernia repair, are all felt to be significant factors.

Despite the relative prevalence and seriousness of recurrent inguinal hernias, there is much cause for encouragement. New methods of diagnosis allow for much more detailed and accurate assessment of hernias than in the past. Recently developed materials, such as polypropylene sutures and synthetic re-enforcing mesh, contribute to greater surgical success than ever before.

A hernia which recurs *should* be repaired. Surgical repair of a recurrent hernia is a more difficult procedure than the initial repair. However, surgeons have addressed the difficulties inherent in a second repair with excellent results.

Techniques have been developed to repair hernias using mesh in sheet, or rolls (plugs). Other surgeons avoid the previous operative site, approach the defect from behind the canal, and insert mesh between the peritoneum and the muscle wall.

Surgeons today enjoy an unprecedented source of information about hernia repair. The wide-spread use of computerization has allowed much more accurate comparison of results of various techniques.

Further, the possibility for medical/surgical specialization has allowed many physicians to take advantage of their greater experience in hernia repair, to the benefit of the patients.

Chapter Six

Femoral Hernias

Since hernias are principally a *structural* problem, certain types occur more frequently to members of one gender (sex) than the other.

The vast majority of hernias in both men and women occur in the *groin* area. They are the result of a weakness in the lower abdominal wall. In males, this is usually an "inguinal hernia". For anatomical reasons, women are much more likely to develop a weakness nearby, called a "femoral hernia".

Characteristics of the femoral hernia include:

1. Greater difficulty in diagnosis

2. Found much more frequently in women

3. Often found in combination with inguinal hernia

4. Usually successfully repaired by one of a variety of surgical approaches

5. Inherent danger of strangulation or incarceration

6. Particularly dangerous to the patient's health

Femoral hernias present real challenges to physicians and surgeons, and create significant risk to the patient.

Some Typical Patients

Femoral hernias are most typically seen in women, These cases include two men and a woman in order to provide a sense of the variety of ways in which patients discover this potentially life-threatening hernia.

"**Tom**" was born in 1910 in a small village near Denham, Massachusetts. His birth was his mother's first, and last, labor. He weighed ten pounds. The doctor performed a forceps extraction and, during the procedure, caused permanent partial paralysis of Tom's right arm.

Now retired, Tom came into the office with a small bulge in his right groin that was only mildly uncomfortable to him as he walked. It disappeared when he lay down. This vague symptom was all that indicated that he had a hernia. Tom's femoral hernia was repaired under local anesthesia. He returned home two hours after surgery and took only minimal pain medication during the week of his recovery. Tom never stopped leading an active lifestyle.

"**Robert**" (83), was severely limited by Parkinson's disease. He suffered from both a tremor and the inability to move about or to urinate easily. He needed moderate assistance from his wife, even when he was feeling his very best. For the two days before he reported to the hospital emergency room (ER), he had nausea and vomiting and was unable to move his bowels. When seen in the ER, Robert's abdomen was distended. An x-ray study showed signs of a bowel obstruction. He also had a very small bulge in his right groin. The bulge was slightly tender and could not be returned to the abdomen, in spite of considerable pressure and maneuvering (it was not reducible). Robert was taken to surgery immediately. He had a small loop of intestine caught in the femoral ring. After reducing the hernia, the intestine was examined. The wall of the intestine was reddish-brown. Robert was given 100% oxygen and the intestine was observed for five minutes; by then the discolored area had turned a healthy pink. With the intestine returned safely to the abdomen, the hernia was repaired and reinforced to help prevent a recurrence. Postoperatively, Robert was quite ill and was in intensive care for four days. His intestine finally regained its normal tone and started to function after the four days. He was in the hospital for another week, in part because of his limited physical ability due to the Parkinson's disease, but also because of the damaged intestine. Robert had no problems with his wound, thanks to the fact there was no contamination from the intestine. **His entire hospital course, however, would probably have been brief if he had received medical attention on the first day of his illness.**

"Sarah" (64) had a moderate mass in her left groin. In fact, it was visibly bulging under her slacks when she came into the office. She had no other symptoms, however, and she noted that the mass decreased in size when she lay down. She was annoyed by the size of the mass and upon examination an incarcerated femoral hernia was found. The hernia was repaired under local anesthesia. Due to the size of the hernia, the inguinal canal and the femoral area were explored. Sarah received "managed anesthesia care" (MAC) during the surgery and went home less than two hours later and had an easy recovery. Because of the type of repair (using special sutures and mesh material), the repaired areas are now extremely strong and resistant to future hernias.

Each of these cases is generally typical, and each enjoyed a successful treatment. However, it is *extremely* important to seek medical attention whenever a hernia is suspected. "Robert's" health was jeopardized by waiting too long to seek help, and both "Tom" and "Sarah" risked possible strangulation of their hernias.

What Makes a Femoral Hernia Unique?

Unlike the more common inguinal hernia, the femoral hernia protrudes below the groin itself and extends into the upper part of the thigh along the route of the blood vessels supplying the legs. There is a small opening at this juncture through which a hernia may develop. Because the blood vessels in this area are called "femoral vessels", the associated hernia has been called a femoral hernia.

Symptoms of a Femoral Hernia

As with most hernias, femoral hernias may present themselves in a variety of ways, from very gradual discomfort to sudden pain. In rare instances, there may be no real discomfort at all. A "bulging" sensation usually accompanies the onset of a femoral hernia and, if swelling in the groin area occurs, the individual should be seen by a physician as soon as possible.

The Anatomy of a Femoral Hernia

A femoral hernia results from the protrusion of abdominal contents through the femoral canal. This canal normally contains the femoral artery and vein as they travel from the abdomen to the thigh in order to supply blood to the leg. **It is the peculiar anatomy of the femoral canal that makes a** femoral hernia extremely dangerous to the patient. One of the four walls of the femoral canal contains a soft vein and artery. The other three walls contain very firm ligaments which are so unforgiving that, once the abdominal contents enter the canal, even modest swelling prevents the hernia from returning normally to the abdominal cavity. See figure 6-A.

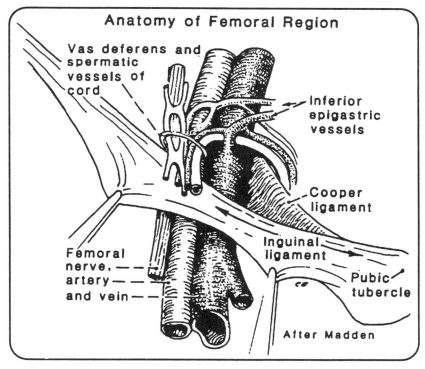

Anatomy of Femoral Region

Vas deferens and spermatic vessels of cord

Inferior epigastric vessels

Cooper ligament

Inguinal ligament

Femoral nerve, artery and vein

Pubic tubercle

After Madden

Figure 6-A

Strangulation tends to occur in a femoral hernia, particularly in older patients. The blood supply to the tissue in the hernia may be pinched, or even shut off completely, by anatomic pressure, and gangrene of the involved tissue may occur. The bladder, fallopian tubes, appendix, colon or omentum (fatty apron of the abdomen), have all been reported as being strangulated in a femoral hernia. **Because of the unusual anatomy of a femoral hernia and the involvement** with the femoral artery and vein, this hernia must be approached with caution. If the intestine is involved and gangrenous, that segment of the intestine must be removed. The intestine is repaired, then replaced into the abdominal cavity.

Problems of Diagnosis of a Femoral Hernia

Many consider the femoral hernia to be difficult for most medical professionals to diagnose. A femoral hernia may enter the thigh, but then flow upward again toward the external inguinal ring, so that both a femoral and inguinal hernia may appear in almost the same area. Figure 6-B shows the close relationship of inguinal and femoral hernias. A direct inguinal hernia is shown, separated by the cord structures. Imagine an indirect inguinal hernia at the same area as the cord, and you will understand the difficulty distinguishing one from the other. There is an extremely small bony prominence on the top of the pubic bone called the "pubic tubercle" (which is about the size of a split pea). If this can be felt, it will usually differentiate the inguinal from the femoral hernia. This is not an easy landmark to find and, occasionally, a femoral hernia patient "appears" to have an inguinal hernia. The femoral canal is also the site of lymphatic drainage from the legs. Therefore, it is

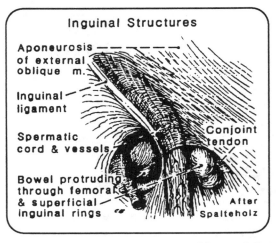

Inguinal Structures

Aponeurosis of external oblique m.

Inguinal ligament

Spermatic cord & vessels

Conjoint tendon

Bowel protruding through femoral & superficial inguinal rings

After Spalteholz

Figure 6-B

possible to have an enlarged lymph node at the femoral canal, further complicating the diagnosis.

Occasionally, a dilated varicose vein may look like a femoral hernia. The femoral hernia can also be so small that it may pinch only a tiny part of the wall of the intestine; this is called a "Richter's hernia". This condition may cause bowel obstruction or even gangrene of the bowel without a noticeable bulge of the femoral canal.

Because of its complex nature, a femoral hernia is among the more difficult medical conditions to accurately diagnose. Even trained medical professionals may have trouble determining the exact cause and extent of involvement. *Accurate self-diagnosis is nearly impossible.*

Causes of a Femoral Hernia

The causes of a femoral hernia are often obscure. These hernias are not related to prenatal development (as the inguinal hernia). They do seem to be related to stress or increased intra-abdominal pressure. **They are more frequently found in women over 40 and there often is a history of repeated pregnancies, chronic cough, or chronic constipation.** Weight loss in the elderly woman may also play a role. The shape of the female pelvis may be an important predisposing factor. The male pelvis is narrow and steep, like a funnel. The female pelvis is broad and shallow, more like a bowl. This bowl-like configuration of the female pelvis may expose the femoral ring in such a manner that the pressures exerted within the abdomen are transmitted more easily toward the femoral canal.

Treatment of a Femoral Hernia

Prompt treatment of a femoral hernia is very important. **Once properly diagnosed, a femoral hernia should be considered for surgical correction.** If incarcerated, the hernia is usually operated on as soon as possible, since serious complications may rapidly develop.

If it is determined that surgery is the best treatment, there are three ways to repair the femoral hernia. **The easiest method is to repair the hernia directly (the "low approach").** The hernia is exposed with an incision directly over the bulge, reduced, and surgically closed. This repair is greatly strengthened by adding polypropylene mesh by one of two methods. One, called the **"umbrella technique"**, consists of the insertion of a circular piece of mesh through the defect. A temporary handle is attached to the midpoint of the circular piece of mesh to facilitate its insertion and orientation, hence the name umbrella. Dr. Bridgman's illustration (figure 6-C) shows the mesh before insertion (above) and during insertion (below). The mesh is then flattened against the superior (upper) entrance to the femoral canal, and the "handle" is then removed.

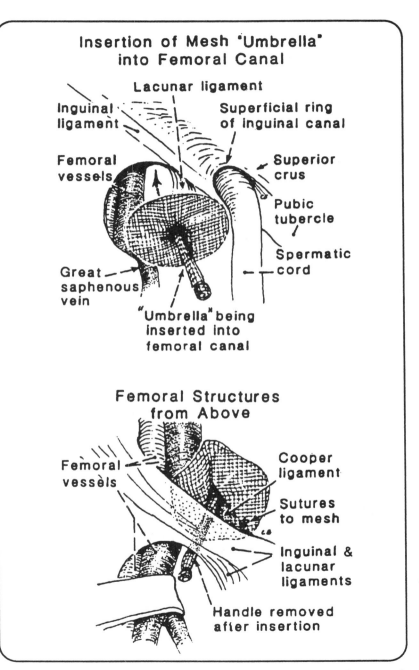

Figure 6-C

The other method known as a **"plug"** consists of a one-inch long roll of mesh which the surgeon prepares during surgery, to fill the defect. See figure 6-D. Both of these methods not only add strength to the repair, but require only a few additional minutes to perform. And most patients seem more comfortable, postoperatively, if mesh is used.

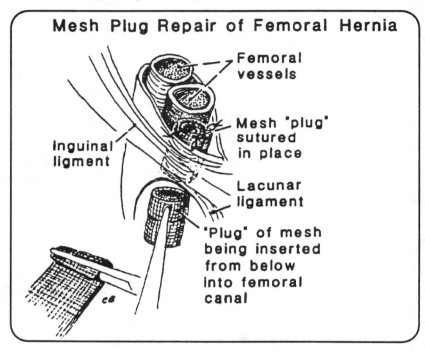

Mesh Plug Repair of Femoral Hernia

Femoral vessels

Mesh 'plug' sutured in place

Inguinal ligment

Lacunar ligament

'Plug' of mesh being inserted from below into femoral canal

Figure 6-D

The second surgical approach is the "inguinal approach". The inguinal canal is exposed in the same manner as to expose and repair an inguinal hernia. However, the femoral ring is then exposed, the hernia is reduced, and both the inguinal and femoral areas are repaired. Mesh or a Goretex® patch may be incorporated into this repair as well.

A third method of repair is the "posterior approach". The inguinal area and the hernia are exposed from behind the abdominal wall. This approach allows for excellent exposure of the area, revealing all of the defects. However, the larger incision, and greater dissection of tissue, makes this a more extensive operation, often requiring post-surgical hospitalization for several days. This approach has been illustrated in Chapter Five.

Typically, the "low approach" is used for most reducible hernias, particularly in the frail patient. It can be performed under local anesthesia and the patient usually is quite comfortable after surgery. The "inguinal approach" is appropriate when there is also an inguinal hernia present, when the hernia is difficult to reduce, or, in those cases where there is a need to define the hernia contents as well as the inguinal anatomy. Local or general anesthesia may be used for this combined approach. Finally, the "posterior approach" may be selected when the hernia is complicated, when there has been a recurrence, or when a bilateral hernia is present. This more complex technique usually requires general or spinal anesthesia.

A femoral hernia should be treated by surgical repair.

What about Anesthesia?

Local anesthetic with MAC is often used in the "low approach" and in the "inguinal approach". If necessary, the local anesthetic may be replaced with general, spinal, or epidural anesthesia, depending on the case. The "posterior approach" usually requires general or spinal anesthesia, since these types of anesthesia produce greater relaxation and optimal control of the operative area. (These topics are discussed in more detail in Chapter Thirteen.) All patients are encouraged to discuss the choice of anesthetic agents with their surgeon and anesthesiologist.

Post-Operative Care

Most femoral hernia treatment is performed on an outpatient basis. Patients arrive at the surgery center about one hour before surgery and are released about one hour after. **By resting and conscientiously applying ice or cold packs to the surgical area, postoperative discomfort and swelling is kept to a minimum.** Generally, a nurse is scheduled to visit the patient at home about six to eight hours after surgery. Additional pain medication can be given at this time (via injection), but seldom is necessary.

Post-surgery office visits are scheduled as indicated by the circumstances, and most patients return to a "careful" normal routine during the first week after surgery.

Some types of surgical repair require a hospital stay which may vary considerably from patient to patient (due to other medical considerations).

Summary

A femoral hernia is often difficult to diagnose, and should almost always be treated by surgical repair. If the hernia is complex or the patient's health is in other ways compromised, hospitalization is usually required. If the femoral hernia is uncomplicated and the repair relatively straightforward, then an outpatient facility is used. Recently introduced techniques with an umbrella or plug of mesh have been used to ease the patient's recovery, while adding strength to the repair. Most patients with a femoral hernia enjoy a comfortable and brief recovery.

A FINAL NOTE:

Femoral hernias should never be ignored!

Chapter Seven

Umbilical Hernias in Infants and Children

Perhaps no emotions are stronger than those of parents for their children. Our protective instincts go into high gear whenever we observe an unusual physical change in our children.

Many parents have been unnerved by the sight of a protruding navel or prominent bulge nearby.

Although potentially serious, umbilical hernias in infants and children are often in fact more difficult for the parents than the child!

How Common Are Umbilical Hernias in Children?

Current studies suggest that umbilical hernias are present in about one-third of all infants *soon after birth*. The incidence seems to be related to birth weight, age and race. In children born prematurely, or with *low* birth weight, the frequency of umbilical hernias is higher: approximately 84% of newborns weighing two to three pounds have an umbilical hernia, as compared to only 21% of those weighing more than five pounds.

Embryonic Development of Umbilical Hernias

While still developing in the uterus, the fetus (called an embryo during the second to the eighth week) obtains its nourishment through large vessels within the "umbilical cord". These vessels attach to the fetus at the midportion of the abdomen (navel, or umbilicus).

Very early in development of the embryo (fourth week), the abdominal wall normally has a very large central "defect" containing intestines. Later, as the embryo develops, the intestines gradually retract into the abdominal cavity, and the size of the defect in the abdominal wall decreases dramatically.

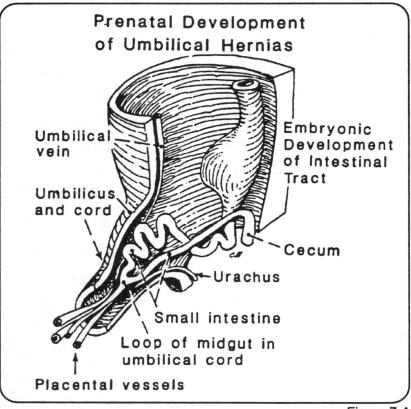

Figure 7-A

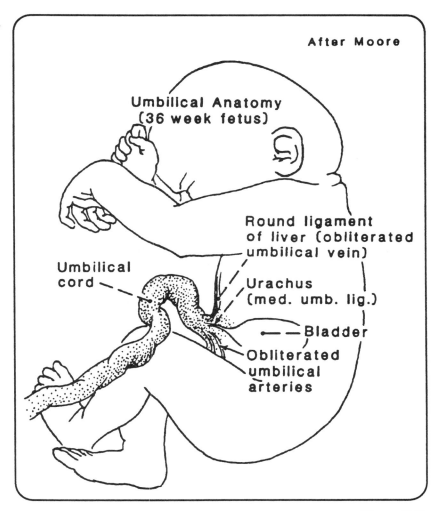

After Moore

Umbilical Anatomy
(36 week fetus)

Round ligament
of liver (obliterated
umbilical vein)

Umbilical
cord

Urachus
(med. umb. lig.)

Bladder

Obliterated
umbilical
arteries

Figure 7-B

At the time of birth, the umbilical defect is just large enough to accommodate the necessary arteries and veins as they pass from the placenta into the infant. When the infant is born, placental circulation stops and these vessels clot. Subsequently, normal scar tissue fills-in the defect in the abdominal wall, and the wall becomes "solid".

The Anatomy of an Umbilical Hernia

An umbilical hernia in an infant or child usually appears as a protrusion of the abdominal tissue through the navel. This typically forms a small sac, which consists of a portion of the abdominal lining (peritoneum). The actual defect in the wall of the abdomen is usually quite small.

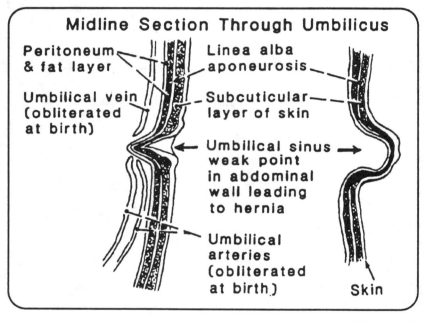

Midline Section Through Umbilicus

Peritoneum & fat layer

Linea alba aponeurosis

Umbilical vein (obliterated at birth)

Subcuticular layer of skin

← Umbilical sinus → weak point in abdominal wall leading to hernia

Umbilical arteries (obliterated at birth)

Skin

Figure 7-C

As a rule, the abdominal contents (or "sac") are easily pushed back into the abdomen with slight finger pressure. The sac may contain abdominal material (such as fat); rarely, it contains intestine.

The abdominal wall consists of multiple muscles that are joined at the midline by canvas-like extensions of the muscle; these extensions are called aponeuroses or fasciae. The term fascia, while not entirely correct, is "easier" to use. Usually, the fascial defect is quite small; although the apparent protrusion of the skin and soft tissue may be large. Careful examination of the fascia in the deep portion of the hernia often reveals only a fingertip-sized defect. The size of the defect is very important, more important than the size of the bulge. A defect in the fascia of less than one inch in diameter will usually close spontaneously. Parents can "feel" this themselves, and its small size may be quite reassuring. It is best to follow the closure of the defect by periodic examination, preferably at monthly intervals. If parents examine the defect more frequently, they may not be able to detect changes because the increments of change will be too small.

An umbilical hernia is easy to diagnose because the protrusion of the navel is very visible. The navel protrudes and expands as the child strains to cry or have a bowel movement, coughs or sneezes.

For a more complete discussion of the anatomy of the abdominal wall and the umbilicus, see the chapter on umbilical hernias in adults.

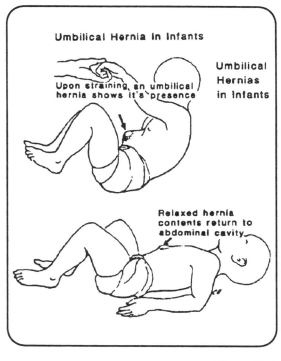

Umbilical Hernia In Infants

Upon straining, an umbilical hernia shows it's presence

Umbilical Hernias in Infants

Relaxed hernia contents return to abdominal cavity

Figure 7-D

What is the Treatment
for an Umbilical Hernia in a Child?

Usually, an umbilical hernia in a child will correct itself with time and require no surgical treatment. Therefore, parents should stay calm and watch and wait. **Almost all small umbilical hernias close spontaneously in the first four years of life.** In one study of 78 patients with umbilical hernias, 31 hernias closed in the first year of life and 72 had closed by the fourth year. If the fascial defect is still larger than about 1/2 inch at age four, the child should be re-evaluated, and surgery may be considered.

Possible Complications

Usually an umbilical hernia can be pushed in with light pressure of the fingertip at the navel, after which the bulge disappears. If the hernia cannot be pushed back into the abdomen, then it is called "incarcerated". When this

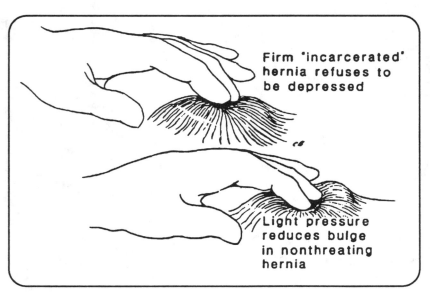

Firm "incarcerated" hernia refuses to be depressed

Light pressure reduces bulge in nonthreating hernia

Figure 7-E

occurs, the tissue inside the hernia swells, the pressure increases, and with time (24 to 48 hours), the tissue becomes gangrenous or dies. An incarcerated hernia is painful to the child and he or she will become unusually "fussy". If the child is in pain and fussing and the hernia cannot be pushed in, you should see your doctor *immediately*. Fortunately, this complication occurs only very rarely.

Another complication, which is often of great concern to the parent, is the breakdown, irritation, or even ulceration of the skin of the protruding navel. However, the probability of this complication occurring is extremely remote. Despite the distortion of the tissue by the hernia, the skin seems to remain healthy with normal hygiene.

A "Grandmother's Remedy"

Sometimes well-intentioned help can provide false information about treating hernias. The phrase "grandmother's remedy" derives from non-professional help that relatives may offer when parents are greatly concerned about their infant or child. One popular grandmother's remedy is placing a 25-cent coin over the hernia and taping it there to prevent protrusion. This effectively corrects the protrusion, but does not cure the

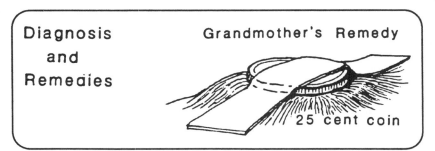

Diagnosis and Remedies

Grandmother's Remedy

25 cent coin

Figure 7-F

hernia. It may even mask a more complicated condition. In short, it is useless.

When to Wait and When to Take Action

It is strongly recommended that parents take a conservative approach to treatment (when the defect is small) because spontaneous correction usually occurs with time and complications rarely occur. If the diameter of the fascial defect is more than one inch, or if the hernia has not closed by the time the child is four years old, the child should be re-evaluated to see if surgery is needed.

If the hernia has not closed by the time the child is ready to go to school (at approximately five years), the psychological embarrassment of the deformity (rather than the physical problems) may suggest treatment.

For example, a seven-year-old boy underwent surgical correction of an umbilical hernia. After surgery, he had some edema (swelling) of the wound. Although the hernia had been satisfactorily closed, the boy was displeased. He was convinced that he had been left with an "outie". He was not convinced that the swelling would go away in a few months. Faced with this situation, approximately ten minutes of cosmetic surgery was performed under local anesthetic to create an "innie" for him. He was then satisfied with the results. This boy's concern illustrates the importance of physical appearance and peer approval at this age.

About Hernia Surgery in Infants and Children

You may wonder what the surgical procedures is like in a child with an umbilical hernia. Surgery is usually performed on children with umbilical hernias in an out-patient facility. A tiny incision is made through the navel and the hernia sac is removed.

Multiple small interrupted sutures help repair the fascial defect and allow the patient's tissue to expand as he or she grows. Polypropylene, a synthetic monofilament material thread, is an ideal suture for this procedure, because it is readily accepted

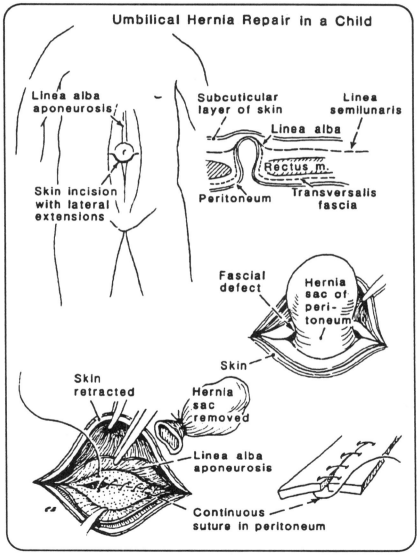

Figure 7-G

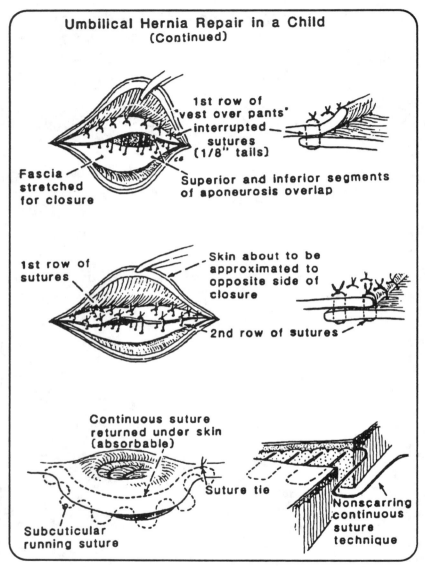

Umbilical Hernia Repair in a Child
(Continued)

1st row of "vest over pants" interrupted sutures (1/8" tails)

Fascia stretched for closure

Superior and inferior segments of aponeurosis overlap

1st row of sutures

Skin about to be approximated to opposite side of closure

2nd row of sutures

Continuous suture returned under skin (absorbable)

Suture tie

Subcuticular running suture

Nonscarring continuous suture technique

Figure 7-H

by the body. New synthetic absorbable sutures are available and are another excellent choice for this repair.

Next, the umbilical skin (which is usually quite thin and may be distended) is fastened to the fascia with delicate temporary sutures to prevent accumulation of fluid after surgery. Finally the incision is closed with absorbable sutures, under the surface. This leaves a nearly invisible scar and eliminates the need to remove any sutures after surgery. A pressure dressing is applied to the wound and should remain in place for a few days if possible. This counteracts (and usually prevents) any post-operative swelling. During the surgery, long-lasting local anesthesia is injected into the wound to prevent post-operative pain.

What About Anesthesia?

Repair of an umbilical hernia in a child proceeds while the patient is sleeping after having received a general anesthetic administered by an anesthesiologist. The child's stomach must be absolutely empty before the administration of the anesthesia, and the child should be in otherwise good health at the time of the surgery. (If the surgery is an emergency procedure because of incarceration or possible gangrene of the hernia, special circumstances may be present.)

The anesthesiologist is well-trained in administering anesthesia to children and should be fully aware of the child's health history, as well as the family's health history. Every effort should be made to have this available at the time of the interview with the anesthesiologist. At that same time, he or she will be pleased to answer any and all questions *you* may have.

Administering general anesthesia does have risks, particularly in children. Great care is taken to reduce or eliminate these risks when surgery is performed.

What About Post-Operative Care?

As a rule, children do not need hospitalization following this surgery. In addition, they do not usually need injections for pain relief, intravenous fluid administration, or prolonged monitoring. Therefore, children are usually treated as out-patients, and are monitored in the recovery room of the out-patient center, and then released to their parents' care. A light diet is recommended during the first 24 hours — clear liquids initially, then diluted milk, then whole milk, and, finally, bland foods. The child can try a regular diet the next day. If a long-lasting local anesthetic has been injected, post-operative discomfort is usually minimal. Usually, over-the-counter medicine (such as Tylenol®) will control any pain that the child may experience at the wound site. Application of ice to the wound area during the first four hours after surgery is extremely important. This, coupled with rest, seems to lessen the tissue's negative reaction to surgery. Usually, an infant or child cannot be forced to lie quietly for a whole day, but an effort should be made to discourage vigorous activity on the day of the surgery. Lots of holding and cuddling is usually effective.

Summary

It is generally best to treat umbilical hernias in infants and children conservatively. A "watch and wait" approach is usually safest for the child. During this period, parents should attend to their infant normally. If the child appears to be in pain or is *unusually fussy*, and the hernia cannot be pushed back into the abdomen with light fingertip pressure, a doctor should be consulted. Otherwise, the hernia typically will correct itself with time. If, after a few years, it is still protruding, the child can be re-evaluated for surgical correction. Surgery, as a rule, is relatively straightforward. Recurrence of this type of hernia is rare.

Chapter Eight

Umbilical Hernias in Adults

Umbilical hernias are relatively common in both adults and children. The navel, or "belly-button", provides a natural weak point in the abdominal wall through which intra- abdominal contents, such as loops of intestine, may pass under pressure.

When thinking of an umbilical hernia in an adult, try to visualize tissue which has been stretched and stretched again, until finally it gives way. Like an overloaded clothes rod in a closet, add one more coat and the rod will give way at its weakest point.

"Typical" Patients

"Sue" can't remember any symptoms of an umbilical hernia until her second pregnancy. She gained a moderate amount of weight and, at about the seventh month of pregnancy, her navel began to protrude.

After her baby was born, she noted with relief that the protrusion had simply disappeared. However, during and after her third pregnancy, the navel protrusion (umbilical hernia) persisted, even when her weight returned to near normal. Finally, the protrusion became about the size of a walnut and didn't seem to reduce in size when Sue would lie down.

"Kenny" is a supervisor for a big-city utility company. As he was loading some heavy equipment, the load shifted and he had to support nearly 200 pounds in order to keep it from falling.

He experienced some pain in his abdomen at the time, but it wasn't until he showered several hours later, that he noticed the protrusion of his navel. Kenny wasn't bothered at first, but when the pain continued, he wisely sought medical attention.

Sue and Kenny represent fairly typical umbilical hernias in adults. Because Sue's weight was in the normal range for her height and build, corrective surgery was successfully completed soon after her diagnosis. Kenny had gained a few pounds annually the past ten years (never enough to cause concern at any one time). He also tended to accumulate this weight in his abdomen, or girth. The fact that he enjoyed two beers nightly may have been important, as well, for this increases the size of the liver by accumulation of fat cells there. All this combined to stretch his abdominal muscles and their canvas-like extensions, fascia. Kenny continued to work, at first. He dieted for six weeks and lost ten pounds. This reduced the tension or tight stretching of his abdominal wall. Then, the hernia was repaired.

Both Sue and Kenny had uneventful convalescences and returned to normal activities in two or three weeks.

Anatomy of an Umbilical Hernia

From a practical standpoint, the anatomy of an umbilical hernia is identical in both children and adults.

Simply put, there is a midline "defect" where the placenta attached to the embryo during fetal development.

The weakness quite often will create a tell-tale protrusion near the navel shortly after birth or during childhood. This frequently will appear to correct itself until circumstances later in life cause its reappearance. It is interesting to note that only about 10 percent of adult patients with umbilical hernias recall having had a navel protrusion as children.

The abdominal wall consists of three fan-like muscles that originate along the sides of the body and "spread-out" until they meet at the midline of the abdomen. Each muscle travels in a different direction, achieving a basketweave effect.

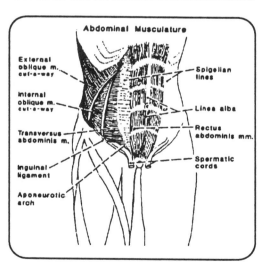

Figure 8-A

Unlike other muscles in the body (which usually end in tendons), the abdominal wall muscles end as a canvas-like material which is properly termed "aponeurosis". For the reader's convenience, this will be called by a more common term, "fascia".

The muscles of each side wrap around and across the abdomen, where the fascia joins at the midline with the fascia of the opposite side. The overall effect is much like that on an elastic girdle.

The union of these muscles *usually* is solid and amazingly strong. However, there may be a weak point or defect anywhere along this seam. When it occurs at the navel, it's known as an umbilical hernia.

To complete a description of the abdominal wall, all of us have large "strap-like" muscles that extend between the chest and the pelvis. These are called "rectus" muscles because they help us to keep our torso vertical when standing or sitting. The pressure of such strong and important muscles unfortunately does *not* help to prevent hernias from occurring, but nevertheless must be carefully considered when planning surgical abdominal wall repair.

The Incidence of Umbilical Hernias in Adults

Several factors seem to effect the development of umbilical hernias in adults: A pre-existing "defect" or untreated childhood hernia; lack of good muscle strength or "tone"; and excess body weight, especially in the stomach area.

Some of these factors can be prevented or altered.

Treatment of an Umbilical Hernia in an Adult

The treatment of an umbilical hernia is dependent upon the size of the hernia, the patient's symptoms, and the actual contents of the hernia (the composition of the material forced through the defect).

Surgical treatment *may* not be necessary, *if:*
1. The hernia is small,
2. The hernia contains only fatty deposits,
3. The hernia is easily pushed back into place (is "reducible").

As the hernia enlarges, or as symptoms such as aching or other discomfort appear, surgical correction usually is recommended.

Fortunately, *most* surgery for umbilical hernias can be scheduled to the patient's convenience; umbilical hernias are rarely life-threatening.

In some rare instances, the hernia cannot be pushed back into the abdomen and is incarcerated. With incarceration, pressure builds *within* the hernia itself, and the blood supply to the hernia's contents is affected. This may lead to tissue death (gangrene), a surgical emergency.

An incarcerated umbilical hernia is *usually* accompanied by significant symptoms, including swelling, soreness or tenderness, and skin discoloration.

Incarceration is 14 times more common in adults than in children.

Since the chances for a small adult umbilical hernia to increase in size (and complexity) are relatively great, anyone suspecting that he or she may have a developing umbilical hernia should seek medical attention. Preventive care is good for your health!

Before any treatment can begin, the hernia must be accurately diagnosed and other related conditions calculated (such as weight, chronic medical conditions, etc.).

Many umbilical hernia patients can benefit from at least *some* weight reduction prior to surgery. This relieves stress of the abdominal wall, allowing muscle tissue to be repaired with less tension. The less tension on the suture line, the better the surgical result.

A Description of the Surgical Procedure

A very small incision is made through the navel, extending only so far as necessary to give adequate access to the hernia site. (Modern surgical instruments allow for much smaller incisions than in years past.)

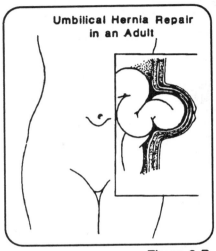

Figure 8-B

The hernia sac is opened and its contents carefully inspected. If there is any portion of the intestine involved, it is inspected and treated as appropriate.

If a strengthening "mesh" is to be used, it is carefully attached between the lining of the abdominal cavity and the overlying fascia. The mesh, when positioned here, is held in place by the abdominal pressure, as well as by the sutures.

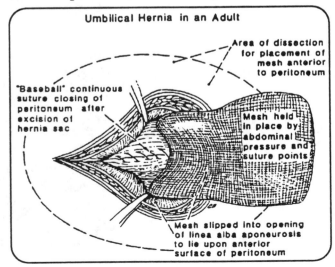

Figure 8-C

The fascia, between the rectus muscles, is then divided transversely with the umbilical defect as the center of the incision. This is then repaired with a suture of polypropylene. Some authors prefer a single layer closure, while others feel more secure with a "vest-over-pants" two layer closure. A running (continuous) suture ('Baseball stitch") distributes the tension evenly throughout the entire suture line.

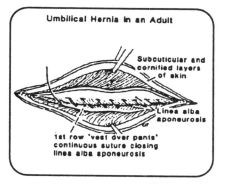

Figure 8-D

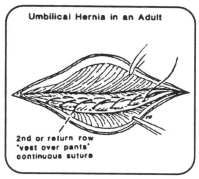

Figure 8-E

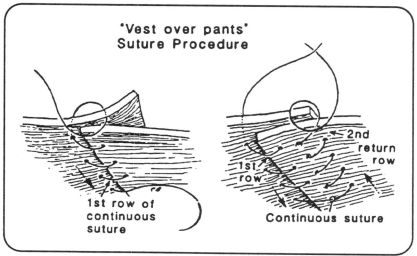

Figure 8-F

The incision is closed with a delicate suture placed under the surface. This technique leaves little if any scar. A pressure dressing is applied to prevent post-operative swelling.

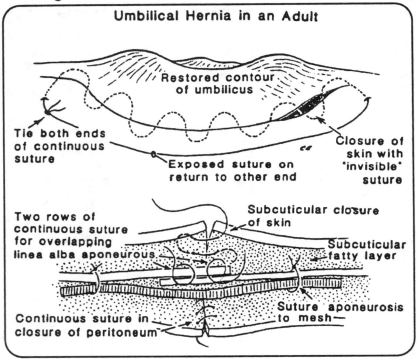

Umbilical Hernia in an Adult

Restored contour of umbilicus

Tie both ends of continuous suture

Exposed suture on return to other end

Closure of skin with 'invisible' suture

Two rows of continuous suture for overlapping linea alba aponeurous

Subcuticular closure of skin

Subcuticular fatty layer

Continuous suture in closure of peritoneum

Suture aponeurosis to mesh

Figure 8-G

Anesthesia

Anesthesia used in umbilical hernia repair varies depending on the patient's age and overall physical condition, the size of the hernia, and the composition of the hernia contents.

Usually, a small hernia can be repaired using only local anesthesia and managed anesthetic care (MAC). The anesthesiologist keeps the patient very comfortable and monitors the general medical condition (heart and respiration, etc.) while the surgeon administers local anesthesia to the surgical area.

The use of long-acting local anesthesia helps to decrease any post-surgical discomfort.

A large hernia may require greater relaxation of the abdominal wall during the repair. Anesthesia methods in these cases include general, spinal or epidural block (please refer to Chapter Thirteen, for more detail).

Post-Operative Care

If the hernia has required a large incision with significant handling of the intestine, the patient may experience a temporary inactivity of the intestines and require intravenous fluids. This mandates hospitalization.

The usual patient, however, does *not* require hospitalization. In most cases, patients return home following surgery, apply ice to the surgical area, rest, and eat a clear liquid diet.

Any post-operative discomfort is controlled with oral medication.

Usually, a nurse is scheduled to visit the patient at home about six to eight hours after surgery. Sutures ("stitches") are removed about a week after surgery and this seldom results in even mild discomfort. Return to normal activities depends upon the extent of the repair and the type of activity usually engaged in.

Ideal surgical hernia repair depends on the skill of the surgeon *and* the common sense of the patient.

Cosmetic Considerations of the Umbilicus

The navel area is cosmetically important. Rod McKuen writes poetry about it. Belly dancing is a cultural art form with the navel as the focus of attention. Pythagoras, the ancient Greek philosopher and mathematician, made a significant observation about human form. He discovered that the navel divides the human body in particular proportions that are pleasing to the general populace. Applying these same proportions in art and architecture resulted in the visual triumphs that continue to delight us today!

Summary

The adult umbilical hernia tends to enlarge with time and frequently becomes more complicated. This form of hernia may be caused by other medical problems, but is often simply the result of excess weight or an enlarged girth.

The hernia, unless it is very small and without other symptoms, should be surgically repaired.

Local anesthesia and out-patient surgery may be sufficient for most umbilical hernias (of "walnut" size or smaller). Some hernias may require general anesthesia and hospitalization.

The umbilicus ("belly-button") has cosmetic value and is restored to its natural appearance whenever possible.

Chapter Nine

Incisional Hernias

An incisional hernia occurs when an organ, or part of an organ, is forced by internal pressure through or along a surgical incision (scar). Such "post-surgical" hernias are relatively rare, and less than half of those patients with an incisional hernia will even recognize the symptoms. Since incisional hernias can be serious, it's important to learn how to identify them.

A "Typical" Case

"Henry" (67), a veteran of World War II, had achieved considerable fame as a photographer. His wartime photos were published nationally, and provided great insight into the challenges and hardships experienced throughout Europe.

Sometimes fate can seem cruel. And so it was with Henry; this most visual of artists was threatened with the loss of his eyesight from illness.

Fortunately, his condition, called temporal arteritis, was identified early and effective intervention begun. Treatment consisted primarily of rather large doses of cortisone, an anti-inflammatory medication. If untreated, Henry would have lost his vision.

Henry also had a history of diverticulitis (inflammation of the abdominal lining), with occasional periods of pain in his left abdomen.

As is often the case with steroid-based medications, the cortisone helped to temporarily mask other symptoms that otherwise would have alerted him to a serious problem.

During a particularly severe episode of diverticulitis, Henry's colon ruptured. This life-threatening condition was finally diagnosed only after it had progressed to include acute peritonitis, or abdominal infection. Emergency surgery saved Henry's life and he seemed to be on the road to recovery.

A word here about "complicated cases". As we grow older, seemingly "minor" complaints can accumulate. As these begin to require treatment, physicians sometimes have to prioritize *which* conditions must be treated first, and which must wait until others are brought under control. This is an excellent reason for treating *any* hernia as soon as possible. In this way, both doctor and patient have the greatest control of treatment.

In the case of Henry, his eye condition took precedence. So, although cortisone is known to sometimes cause healing problems, its administration was continued before and after surgery. Consequently, it was little surprise that Henry developed a hernia along the new incision line created by his emergency surgery.

Since the hernia could be managed, its treatment was postponed until his eye condition cleared up enough to stop the cortisone without endangering his sight.

About a year later, surgical repair of the hernia was completed, using polypropylene mesh to assure the strongest possible final result.

Although Henry's situation may seem a little extreme, it actually represents a relatively common scenario; incisional hernias frequently appear in patients whose surgical healing is compromised by any of a number of other factors, from excess weight to chronic coughing.

Incidence of Incisional Hernias

Incisional hernias occur in about two to ten percent of *abdominal* surgery patients. This figure varies according to the specific type of surgery, as well as the patient's individual condition.

Location of Incisional Hernias

Incisional hernias tend to occur wherever the incision is made. Please remember, surgeons frequently do not have a good choice of incisional placement. Most incision placement is dictated by the underlying condition.

Hernias tend to occur where the nerves or the circulation to the area has been compromised. To illustrate, an incision, laterally under the rib cage margin, may interrupt the nerves which supply the triangle of skin and muscle from the incision to the midline. Any subsequent incision in that triangle may develop a hernia in the second incision. Similarly, any incision placed near and parallel to another vertical scar may develop a hernia.

Many old-style abdominal operations (such as those for gallbladder removal or appendectomy) inherently created increased incisional hernia risk. Those procedures have been refined to *greatly* reduce the causes of incisional hernias associated with them.

An incisional hernia is most likely to appear along a *vertical*, midline incision (chest to navel). Such an incision can take up to 120 days to heal. Any injury to the incision or to the patient during this time may contribute to the creation of an incisional hernia.

Naturally, this type of incision is avoided whenever possible, but since it allows for rapid access in cases of emergency and the greatest exposure of the inner abdomen, it sometimes is essential. Many cases *must* be explored using a vertical midline incision, despite increased risk of incisional hernia.

Symptoms of an Incisional Hernia

Usually, a visible bulge will appear beneath the incision scar. This "bump" is softer and more pronounced than the scar tissue, and can be felt by hand. Frequently, the overlying skin is quite healthy and well-healed. Most patients notice that the bulge (hernia) increases with coughing or straining. When the patient reclines, the hernia may seem to disappear.

Often, the hernia actually consists of multiple openings, and the total area of involvement is nearly always considerably larger than the visible bulge.

It is usually practical to proceed directly with surgery and to define any existing or potential defects. If there are pre-operative questions about the size and location of the hernia, we are fortunate to have ultrasound available to diagnose the problem pre-operatively. This study determines the exact size and location of the fascial defects.

Again, only about 40 percent of patients with an incisional hernia will complain of noticeable symptoms. In rare cases a loop of intestine (bowel) is caught in the hernia gap. When this occurs, the patient typically becomes nauseated and may have abdominal cramps or vomiting.

If the loop of intestine is involved in the hernia, and is sufficiently kinked, the patient may be unable to pass digested products out of the body. Ignoring a seemingly "minor" hernia may lead to other problems.

If the hernia is allowed to become large, the overlying skin may become irritated or even ulcerated.

Many patients discover the incisional hernia when they bend over or twist, or are otherwise active. Still others seek medical attention because of embarrassment over the bulge's unsightly appearance. Though embarrassment is unnecessary, *accurate diagnosis and treatment is vital!*

Causes of an Incisional Hernia

Incisional hernias may occur anywhere in the abdomen wherever surgery has taken place. Larger incisions, incisions that involve wide exposure of the abdomen (i.e., vertical midline incisions), and incisions that may damage or even destroy nerve supply to the abdominal wall are more prone to develop hernias.

Approximately 60 percent of patients who develop incisional hernias have an infection within the abdomen at the time of their operation. This infection may be the result of an abscess, a ruptured bowel (such as with acute appendicitis or a ruptured diverticulum), or from more general inflammatory bowel disease.

Patients undergoing treatment with steroids have a higher incidence of hernia formation (a warning to bodybuilders or athletes), because steroids can interfere with the healing process.

Obesity (in excess of 15 percent over ideal weight) is also a frequent contributing factor, due to the extra strain and pressure on the incision.

Less common causes of an incisional hernia are age (over 40), anemia, malnutrition, diabetes, and post-operative intestinal obstruction resulting in excess pressure.

Post-operative *chest* infections are associated with an increased incidence of hernia formation.

Of particular concern, and one of the few *preventable* factors, is smoking. Patients who smoke often have a chronic cough and compromised ability to clear secretions from the lungs. Patients who smoke are frequent victims of an incisional hernia.

The suture material that is used in the original surgery may also be a contributing factor to the incidence of an incisional hernia. Some sutures are absorbable and may dissolve before the wound has attained its maximum strength. Other sutures (such as silk) are woven and these porous sutures may harbor bacteria within their fibers. Later, stitch abscesses may form and wound breakdown may follow.

This subject is covered more completely in Chapter Five, Recurrent Inguinal Hernias.

Treatment of Incisional Hernias

As with most hernias, the preferred treatment for incisional hernias is via permanent, surgical repair. Timing is crucial. If the hernia is small, it can usually be repaired with ease. If there is undue delay, the hernia may grow and the surgery become more difficult.

Obviously, it is important to eliminate any causative factors *before* repairing the hernia. It may be preferable (or necessary) to wait until excess weight has been lost, coughing (such as from uncontrolled asthma) has been controlled, and certainly until any known infection has been eliminated. In the case of infection, a delay of six to twelve months is common.

It is highly recommended that smokers stop smoking at least two months prior to surgical repair of an incisional hernia and not smoke for at least four months following.

Surgery of Incisional Hernias

The body's normal anatomy is retained or reconstructed whenever possible. In order to maximize incision strength, permanent suture material is used. An effort is made *not* to disturb, expose or manipulate the intestine during the operation, for this may cause a temporary loss of bowel tone with resultant abdominal distention and discomfort.

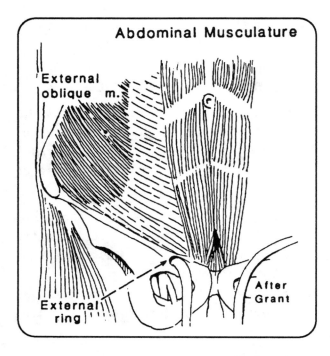

Abdominal Musculature

External oblique m.

External ring

After Grant

Figure 9-A

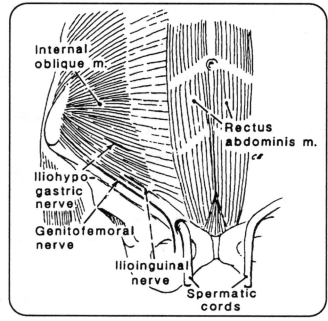

Internal oblique m.

Rectus abdominis m.

Iliohypo-gastric nerve

Genitofemoral nerve

Ilioinguinal nerve

Spermatic cords

Figure 9-B

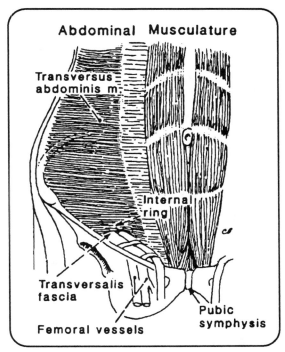

Figure 9-C

Figures 9-A, 9-B, and 9-C illustrate the normal anatomy of the abdominal wall.

Incisional hernias result from a breech in this anatomy. A repair must attempt to restore the normal anatomical relationships.

The hernia should be repaired with a minimum of tension. If there is tension on the suture line, the sutures and tissues may be weakened during the post-operative period. If it is not possible to repair the tissues without tension, a prosthetic material, such as polypropylene mesh, is inserted which will usually hold the incision's edges in an optimal position.

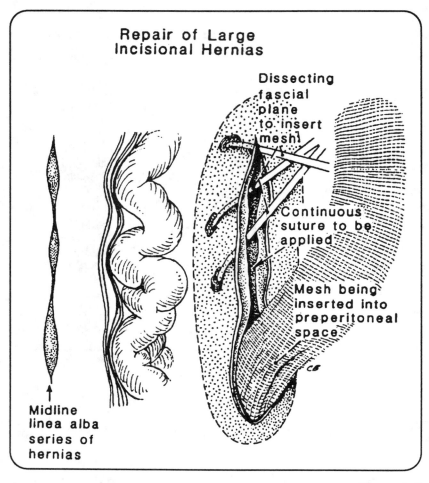

Repair of Large Incisional Hernias

Dissecting fascial plane to insert mesh

Continuous suture to be applied

Mesh being inserted into preperitoneal space

Midline linea alba series of hernias

Figure 9-D

It is preferable not to use mesh in an *infected* area, but occasionally there is no satisfactory alternative. Polypropylene mesh has the surprising characteristic of almost always healing without additional complications, even in infected areas.

Since extensive surgical dissection may be required when repairing an incisional hernia, large areas of tissue have to be separated from one another and drains are usually inserted. These drains are left in place for a few days to prevent the accumulation of fluid. The involved tissue (between fascia and skin) is often closed with multiple fine absorbable sutures in an attempt to avoid a collection of fluid at the surgical site. The incision is closed with sutures or clips. A variety of techniques is used to achieve the best possible cosmetic result.

About Pneumoperitoneum

Pneumoperitoneum (new-mo-peri-toe-neum) simply means "air within the abdomen".

When used in connection with hernia surgery, pneumoperitoneum describes a technique of gently introducing air into the abdomen to expand the abdominal wall prior to the repair of an incisional hernia.

Small amounts of air are injected (using local anesthetic) into the abdominal cavity two or three times weekly, prior to surgery. This expansion enlarges the abdominal wall.

At the time of surgery, the air is removed and the enlarged abdominal wall then has more slack in it, which allows for a more tension-free repair. As described earlier, too much tension can interfere with proper healing, with proper function of the diaphragm, and may even contribute to a recurrence of the hernia.

Summary

Incisional hernias develop in a relatively small percentage of abdominal surgery patients.

Some contributing factors to incisional hernias can be controlled, but such hernias frequently are the result of *necessary* incision placement.

Incisional hernias rarely are incarcerated (or "strangulated") but do tend to enlarge with time and should be surgically repaired as soon as practical.

Before repair of an incisional hernia, every effort should be made to correct any factors that may have contributed to the causes of the hernia. These same factors, such as obesity, or chronic coughing, may cause a *recurrence* of the hernia.

Successful incisional hernia repair requires surgical reconstruction of the natural abdominal wall anatomy, with as little suture tension as possible.

New techniques and materials have greatly improved both the comfort and success of incisional hernia repair.

Chapter Ten

Hernias of the Diaphragm

As with many medical conditions, hernias of the diaphragm and related structures come in several varieties. Fortunately, they are generally easier to understand than to pronounce!

About the Diaphragm.

Simply stated, the diaphragm is a muscular wall separating the abdomen (stomach area) from the thoracic cavity (chest).

Remembering that a hernia occurs when any organ or part of an organ protrudes through the wall of the cavity that normally contains it, the most common diaphragmatic hernias are:

- Hiatus hernia. This must be evaluated and treated separately from gastroesophageal reflux disease (GERD)
- Paraesophageal hernia
- Congenital diaphragmatic hernia
- Traumatic diaphragmatic hernia

What is a Hiatus Hernia?

The majority of patients with a hernia of the diaphragm in fact have a hiatus hernia. In simplified terms, when a portion of the stomach is displaced, or pushed, through the normal opening of the diaphragm wall, we call it a hiatus hernia.

A hiatus hernia, because it is contained by the abdomen and chest cavity, is never felt as a lump. It usually is discovered because of discomfort. Hiatus hernias may become strangulated, but this is extremely rare.

Usually, the lowest part of the esophagus (the tube-like organ through which food and secretions pass from the mouth and throat to the stomach) joins the stomach just below the diaphragm wall. This allows food to pass easily into the stomach. The esophagus must penetrate the diaphragm as it travels into the abdominal cavity. There is a normal opening in the diaphragm muscle which is just large enough for the esophagus. This opening is called a hiatus.

The joining of the esophagus and stomach includes a natural valve-like mechanism that prevents the contents of the stomach from regurgitating (or returning to) the esophagus. This is called the lower esophageal sphincter (LES).

Nature's marvelous design allows us to eat, swallow and transport food to the stomach, even while engaged in physical activity (remember the last time you grabbed a snack "on the run"?). In some people, however, the lower esophagus may find a way to rise above the diaphragm, through an enlargement of the normal diaphragm passageway or "diaphragmatic hiatus", and into the chest cavity. When this happens, the uppermost portion of the stomach may be pulled along with it. The causes of this movement are many and varied — from the aging process to an imbalance of internal pressure.

Often the hiatus hernia is quite small. In most cases, patients have a hiatus hernia and don't even know it! In fact, the majority of people over 50 years old may have a minor hiatus hernia.

The "Sliding" Hiatus Hernia

When the hiatus hernia involves the movement of the esophagus and connected stomach up into the chest cavity, we call it a "sliding" hiatus hernia.

A sliding hiatus hernia may come and go, depending upon the body's position (i.e., reclining), the content level within the stomach, and other factors. This is the most common form of all diaphragmatic hernias.

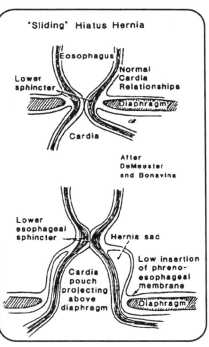

Figure 10-A

About Gastroesophageal Reflux Disease (GERD)

Since you now know that most people with a simple hiatus hernia are seemingly free of symptoms, you also should know that a moderate number of patients will complain of heartburn, or reflux of their stomach contents into the esophagus, yet not have a hiatus hernia! Gastroesophageal reflux disease (GERD) is the technical term for this regurgitation and resultant discomfort. Patients often describe belching of gas which feels like a "red hot poker"; therefore the term, *heartburn*.

Heartburn occurs because the chemicals found naturally in the stomach (including potent hydrochloric acid and the enzyme pepsin) cause severe irritation and inflammation of the esophagus. The lining of the stomach is tolerant of acid, and resists its effect; the esophagus is not.

When the stomach, for whatever reason, forces stomach acid into the esophagus, most people complain of a burning, hot sensation in the middle of their chest, behind the breastbone. In addition to acid and pepsin, other contents (including bile) may offend. But, since acid and pepsin are nearly always present, the condition is sometimes referred to as "peptic esophagitis".

It is important to understand that GERD, or "heartburn", is not a necessary consequence of a hiatus hernia. It is also true that GERD may occur when no hiatus hernia is present.

What is the Treatment for a Hiatus Hernia?

A hiatus hernia is treated only if it is symptomatic, as evidenced by "heartburn" or GERD. Both the diagnosis and the treatment of this condition are usually managed medically, rather than surgically. Medical treatment is effective in 80 to 90 percent of those with noticeable symptoms. *After the diagnosis has been established*, the general measures of therapy are as follows:

Treatment You Can Do for Yourself

A. Mechanical intervention to reduce reflux.

1. *Lose weight*, if you are overweight. The loss of even a few pounds often produces dramatic relief. Your abdomen, if protuberant in a standing position, flattens out when you lie down, thus pressing the abdominal contents into the chest.

2. *Elevate the head of your bed*. Some patients prefer sleeping in a reclining chair or a special bed or mattress that elevates the upper half of the bed. Some physicians recommend that the head of the bed be elevated on eight-inch blocks. Occasionally, many large pillows may provide adequate elevation.

3. *Avoid eating any food three hours before reclining*. Many patients also notice improvement when they change their heaviest meal from evening to mid-day.

B. Modify Your Diet.

1. Avoid foods that relax the valve-like action of the lower esophageal sphincter (LES). The list includes fat, chocolate, alcohol, and peppermint. Fat is the worst offender!

2. Avoid foods that tend to produce gas. These distend the stomach and thereby increase GERD.

3. Avoid foods that directly irritate the esophagus, such as citrus, colas and most other sodas, as these are very acidic. Coffee also irritates the esophagus.

C. **Stop smoking.** Cigarettes, or nicotine products, act by relaxing the lower esophageal sphincter (LES) and by stimulating stomach acid secretion. If complete abstinence isn't possible, it is essential to refrain from smoking whenever reclining and before retiring (sleeping).

D. **Consider using lozenges at night.** Some physicians recommend that patients use lozenges. When the patient sleeps, saliva, which moistens and neutralizes the mouth and esophagus, is secreted in decreased amounts. Lozenges stimulate the flow of saliva and this helps protect the esophagus during sleep.

E. **Avoid use of medications which are known irritants** to the stomach. This includes aspirin and the other anti-inflammatory drugs such as you would take for arthritis.

F. **Use antacids.** Antacids are medicines which are taken by mouth and are available, over the counter, at drug stores. Liquid antacids are more effective than tablets. The liquid coats the lining of the esophagus and stomach and protects the lining from the acid. Brand names include Maalox®, Gelusil®, and Titralac®. Gaviscon® is particularly valuable, as it is an antacid in a foam which forms a protective cap at the junction of the stomach and esophagus.

It should be recognized that there can be side effects from the long term use of antacids. These can include diarrhea (or constipation, depending on the brand), altered calcium metabolism, and magnesium retention. As with other symptoms, if prolonged use of antacids seems necessary, *a physician should be consulted*.

Medical Treatment Your Doctor Might Prescribe

A. Reduce Gastric Acid Secretion.

Prescription of "H2-receptor" blocking agents. These are medications which reduce the amount of acids created by the stomach. These are prescription drugs. Brand names include Tagamet®, Zantac®, and Pepcid®, and Axid®

B. Evaluate your medications and consider elimination of drugs which decrease LES. This includes medication which have a sedative effect, such as some sleeping pills, muscle relaxants, such as Librax®, Bentyl®, and Donnatal®. You will probably have to ask your doctor about these. Other drugs which decrease LES, such as medications for hypertension, medications such as Procardia® for your heart, and Amantadine® for Parkinsonism, MUST be discussed with your doctor.

C. Prescription of drugs which stimulate the LES muscle tone. Reglan® is used for this purpose, but must be used with caution.

D. Prescription of Prilosec®. Prilosec®, a newly developed medication, is an even more potent inhibitor of stomach acid secretion than the H2-receptor blocking agents listed above. This drug is used in patients who have cooperated with all of the preceding treatment plan, yet continue to have symptoms. This drug is especially effective. Its long term effects are not yet known. The medical profession tends to restrict use of new medications until animal testing and prolonged patient use have been proven to be safe as well as successful.

What If Medical Treatment Fails?

Surgical correction of hiatus hernias is considered for the *small* percentage of patients who have failed to respond to the above treatment plan. There are numerous surgical procedures available. These operations are major surgery, however, and are not entered into lightly.

The Rudolph Nissen fundoplication, an awkward sounding treatment introduced in 1951, consists essentially of surgically relocating the upper portion of the stomach from its normal position just under the diaphragm, and wrapping it around the esophagus at its lowest point. This attempts to recreate the valve-like juncture between the esophagus and the stomach, allowing food to enter the stomach, but not return into the esophagus.

Another popular procedure is the Hill procedure, first advocated by Lucius Hill, M.D., in 1967. This is also performed through the abdominal incision. The operation returns the stomach back down into the abdomen, and attempts to reconstruct the juncture of the esophagus to the stomach so that the valve-like action is restored. The muscles of the diaphragm are sutured, tightening the hiatus.

There is a modification of the Nissen procedure which is performed through the chest wall, and this is used when the esophagus is short, preventing the return of the stomach into its normal abdominal position.

There is another operation performed through the chest called a Belsey Mark IV procedure, which also repairs the diaphragm. There is even a prosthesis called the "Angelchik" that is designed to be surgically placed around the esophagus at its junction with the stomach in order to recreate the valve-like action between the esophagus and stomach.

It should be reassuring to the patient that so many surgical procedures are available. Though no one technique is universally effective, surgical correction of a hiatus hernia is generally successful.

The Paraesophageal Hiatal Hernia

Although relatively rare (and very difficult to pronounce!), the paraesophageal hiatal hernia is none-the-less *quite serious*.

This is a hernia, through the wall of the diaphragm, **immediately adjacent to the opening for the esophagus** (See figure 10-B). Paraesophageal hiatal hernias occur in approximately five percent of the patients with a hiatal hernia. This condition, in contrast to the hernias in the previous discussion, is nearly always treated surgically, for it is life-threatening approximately 20 percent of the time.

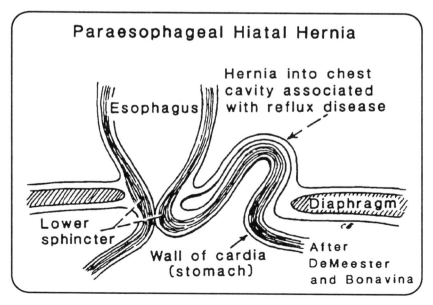

Figure 10-B

The patient may complain of few, if any, symptoms. Therefore, the symptoms may appear to be quite similar to those of a patient with hiatus hernia or reflux peptic esophagitis. Other patients may seem to suffer with ulcers and bleeding, or even signs of obstruction to the stomach. Occasionally, there is a severe abdominal catastrophe. Here, there is a sudden "torsion" or twisting of the stomach that is so severe that the blood supply to the stomach is obstructed. This can result in gangrene of the stomach wall. When gangrene does occur, the patient experiences sudden severe pain.

The high potential for life-threatening complications nearly always demands surgical intervention.

In order to be certain that the hernia is, in fact, a paraesophageal hiatal hernia, diagnostic studies, including x-rays (with swallowed barium) and gastroscopy, are usually performed.

Surgery to Correct Paraesophageal Hiatal Hernia

The surgical correction of this problem depends primarily on its presentation. If the patient is not in acute distress, and preoperative evaluation is permitted, studies such as esophageal pressure measurements and 24-hour esophageal PH (acid test) allow the physician to determine if there is adequate valve-like action between the esophagus and stomach. If the valve-like action can be demonstrated before surgery, the operation can be simplified. The stomach is simply returned into the abdominal cavity and the diaphragm defect is sutured; additional surgery, such as the Nissen procedure is not needed.

If the stomach has become gangrenous, the surgeon has no choice but to remove the entire stomach, repair the defect in the diaphragm and re-establish continuity of the esophagus to the digestive tract.

With paraesophageal hiatal hernia, the degree of seriousness is directly related to the extent to which the stomach has migrated through the diaphragm, into the chest cavity. Most are discovered early enough that life-threatening complications are avoided.

What is a Congenital Diaphragmatic Hernia?

Occasionally, infants are born with a defect in the diaphragm, particularly on the left side, and located toward the back of the diaphragm. This results from a failure of development in the embryo during the third to ninth week. The prognosis for survival, after surgical repair of this diaphragm defect, is often divided into two categories.

1. Patients where the defect is noted during the first 24 hours immediately following birth. These patients often have marked underdevelopment of the lung on that same side of the chest. This limits the number of survivors.

2. Patients where the defect is noted after the first 24 hours following birth. Here, the lungs are significantly more developed and, therefore, utilize inhaled oxygen much more effectively. In this case, there is enhanced infant survival.

Congenital diaphragmatic hernias are usually treated by pediatric surgeons.

There is another defect, which sometimes occurs in the diaphragm immediately adjacent to the sternum, or breastbone. This is called a "hernia of Morgagni". It usually is smaller, and is often found late in life. The hernia of Morgagni enjoys a reputation as "easy to repair". The hernia opening is small. It is easily exposed through an abdominal incision. The defect is easily repaired. And, the risk to the patient is low.

Medical and surgical conditions affecting infants and children (and, today, the unborn), always are particularly sensitive. Fortunately, great strides continue to be made in the treatment of our youngest patients.

What is a Traumatic Diaphragmatic Hernia?

Occasionally, with crushing injuries, such as experienced in high speed traffic and job-site injuries, the force of the blow to the abdomen is so great that the diaphragm is torn or ruptured, usually on the patient's left side. During the same accident, there frequently are many other injuries to the patient, such as broken bones and injuries to the intra-abdominal contents. **These diaphragmatic tears are usually relatively easily repaired, if diagnosis can be effectively made in the face of other, often more pressing, complications.** Even x-rays obtained in a trauma situation are frequently inadequate because of the multiple problems involved.

Often the trauma surgeon is faced with other overwhelming injuries which must take precedence. And, because this injury may be "silent", it is occasionally not discovered until one to three days later. Then, a routine chest x-ray will be taken and will reveal that intestine has been displaced into the chest cavity to lie alongside the lung.

Few areas of medicine have benefited from such rapid advancements as trauma care. New diagnostic techniques, including computer assisted tomography (CAT scans), magnetic resonance imaging (MRI) and sonography provide emergency medical personnel with information undreamed of only a decade ago. With the addition of more sophisticated life-saving medications and procedures, the trauma victim has a better chance of survival and recovery than ever before. And, as the patient's overall prognosis improves, so does the outlook for repair of a traumatic diaphragmatic hernia.

Summary

Hiatus hernias (involving the diaphragm) are primarily a medical condition. Frequently they are not symptomatic. If there is gastro-esophageal reflux disease (GERD) that is symptomatic with heartburn and fails to respond to medical treatment, surgery may be considered. Fortunately, there is much that the patient can do to help.

There are numerous surgical procedures that have been developed to correct gastroesophageal reflux.

Paraesophageal diaphragmatic hernias are rare. These are treated surgically, since approximately one-fifth of the patients may experience a life-threatening situation. It is extremely important to differentiate the simple hiatus hernia, the gastroesophageal reflux (reflux peptic esophagitis), and the paraesophageal hernia.

Congenital defects of the diaphragm are repaired surgically. These often are associated with other birth defects.

A traumatic hernia of the diaphragm may occur with high speed auto accidents and industrial injury. These are repaired surgically. They are frequently associated with other severe injuries.

Clearly, there is much that can be done to correct the discomfort and potential danger of diaphragmatic hernias.

Doctors are always working to preserve our health and cooks to destroy it, but the latter are the more often successful.

Denis Diderot, (1713-1784)

Chapter Eleven

Unusual Hernias

There are a number of hernias that are *relatively* uncommon. These include:

Epigastric hernia
Spigelian hernia
Lumbar hernia
Obturator hernia
Pelvic floor hernia
Internal hernia

Though less common than other types, these hernias nonetheless can cause considerable discomfort and *may* be life-threatening. As with nearly all hernias, surgery is generally recommended as the preferred treatment. Just as with the more common types of hernia, modern surgical techniques make repair much easier for the patient than continuing to live with a bothersome and perhaps dangerous condition.

Epigastric Hernias

The term "epigastric" refers to the upper and middle of the abdomen, or to the linea alba. Epigastric hernias occur at the middle of the abdominal wall, between the umbilicus and the lower chest. They are found in approximately 2% of the population and are slightly more common in males. Epigastric hernias are rarely seen in children.

Anatomy

Epigastric hernias result in a small, but sharply outlined, defect in the linea alba. The crisscross pattern of the three lateral abdominal muscles, which extend across the rectus muscles and the midline, allows for movement, yet is extremely strong. However, in some cases, a weak point may occur, allowing the abdominal organs and tissue to pass through the abdominal wall. (See figures 9-A, 9-B, and 9-C in Chapter Nine, page 118.) These illustrate the extensions from each of the lateral abdominal muscles. These extensions continue around the rectus muscles, then cross the midline and contribute to the tissue strength for a considerable distance on the other side, as well. (See figure 4-C, page 35.)

The causes of such defects aren't well known. Some researchers feel that an epigastric hernia develops because of a weakness associated with the blood vessels and nerve fibers as they pass through the muscles. Others report that *most* epigastric hernias occur because the fascial structure is deficient.

Symptoms

About 75% of patients complain of pain from an epigastric hernia. Usually intermittent, the pain often is severe and out of proportion to the associated visible bulge.

Epigastric hernias nearly always protrude visibly, and may range from pea-sized to as large as a football.

Presentation of an Epigastric Hernia

These hernias almost always protrude in the midline, but may also deviate away from the midline, extending superficially, into the rectus muscle area. In these cases, the diagnosis is less obvious. They may even be misdiagnosed as tumors.

Treatment of an Epigastric Hernia

Treatment is usually conservative in children less than four years of age. One study followed a series of children between the ages of two to seven years and found that epigastric hernias resolved spontaneously with time in the majority of these patients. The decision for surgery in children depends on the symptoms of the hernia and its size, allowing nature to heal the hernia if it is small and free of symptoms.

Surgery is recommended for adults if the hernia is painful or if the fascial defect is greater than a fingertip diameter.

Recurrence

Recurrence of this type of hernia is rare. However, healing is very slow (approximately four months), and the patient should be very guarded in his or her activities for the post-operative period.

Spigelian Hernias

This is a very rare hernia that usually occurs at the belt line. There have been 744 cases reported in the most recently available literature. All ages have been reported, from 6 to 94.

Anatomy of a Spigelian Hernia

The transverse muscle of the abdomen converts to a fascial or aponeurotic extension at the lateral border of the rectus muscle, as the rectus muscle extends from the chest wall to the pubis. This transition was first described by the famous anatomist, Adrian Van der Spieghle. Dr. Van der Spieghle described the muscle structure as the "linea semilunaris", because of its curvature as it extended from chest to pelvis. Anatomists converted Dr. Van der Spieghle's name to the Latin form. Subsequently, any hernia which developed in this line was known as a Spigel's or Spigelian hernia.

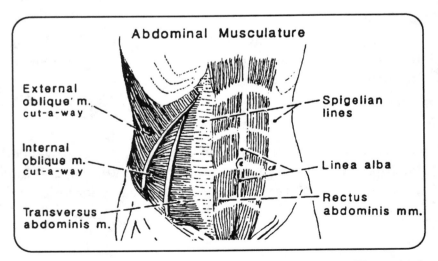

Figure 11-A

By definition, any hernia that occurs in Spigel's fascia (see figure 11-A) is a Spigel's hernia. It is also true that Spigel's hernias are found throughout the length of the abdomen, and it is not unusual to have a Spigel's hernia misdiagnosed as a direct inguinal hernia. The most common location, however, is at the beltline.

Clinical Characteristics

Incarceration at the time of surgery occurs about 20% of the time.

In a few cases, the hernia sac may present under the skin, but usually the hernia is located between the muscles and their aponeurotic extensions in the anterior abdominal wall. In these latter cases, a mass is frequently not apparent. These patients usually complain of discomfort in the area where the sac is caught in the muscle wall.

Diagnosis of a Spigelian Hernia

A bulge is frequently not apparent, making diagnosis difficult. Discomfort or pain in the area is a common presenting complaint. Diagnosis is then made by clinical suspicion, tenderness in the area, and *confirmation* with either an ultrasound study or CAT scan. Entrapped anterior skin nerves of thoracic vertebrae levels 10, 11, and 12 may produce discomfort resembling Spigelian hernias. A thorough knowledge of the anatomy of the area is essential.

Treatment of a Spigelian Hernia

Treatment of a Spigelian hernia is surgical. Once the diagnosis has been established, the area is explored and repair is relatively straightforward. Local anesthesia is ideal for the repair of these hernias when they are small. The results of surgery for Spigelian hernias are excellent and recurrences are infrequent.

Lumbar Hernia

A lumbar hernia consists of a hernia in the flank, located in the midlevel of the back, halfway between the midline and the lateral margin of the back. These hernias must be differentiated from fatty tumors (lipomas), tumors of the muscle or fascia, hematomas (collections of blood), abscesses and kidney tumors.

Anatomy

Lumbar hernias are divided into two types:

1) The "inferior lumbar" hernia is named after Jean Louis Petit, who first described it in the early 1700's. This hernia is located immediately over the crest of the pelvic bone.

2) The "superior lumbar" hernia was first described by Grynfeltt in 1855. This hernia is found in a

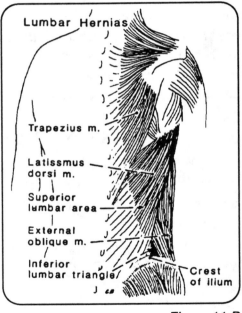

Figure 11-B

quadrangle in the lumbar area, which is covered by the latissimus dorsi muscle. Because of this coverage, the bulge of the hernia may be masked.

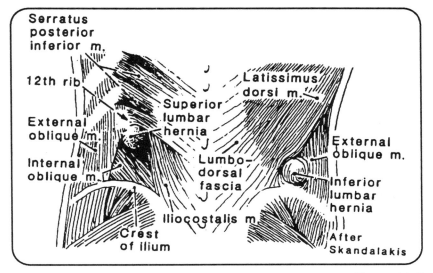

Figure 11-C

Treatment

Lumbar hernias rarely result in strangulation, and therefore the prognosis is good. They do gradually increase in size, however, and may become symptomatic and cosmetically displeasing. The surrounding muscles become deformed due to stretching and become more difficult to repair. For these reasons, *early surgical correction is recommended.*

Obturator Hernia

An obturator hernia protrudes from the abdominal cavity through the pelvis into the thigh. The defect is located deep to the femoral area at the groin juncture. It rarely creates a bulge that can be felt by the physician. Occasionally, there is a small area of discoloration noted on the skin over the region. Therefore, a hernia is often not suspected because of this absence of physical signs. The patient usually develops symptoms of a bowel obstruction and diagnosis is not made until an exploratory abdominal operation is performed and the bowel is found to be kinked within the obturator opening.

The location of an obturator hernia is illustrated in figure 11-D. A view of the same area from *inside* the pelvis is seen in figure 5-C, page 71.

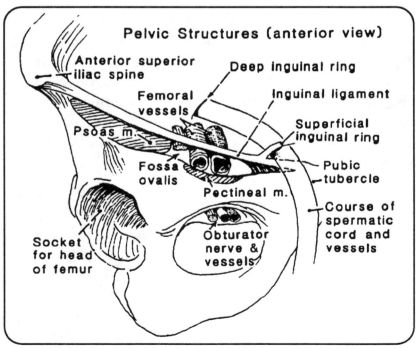

Pelvic Structures (anterior view)

Anterior superior iliac spine

Deep inguinal ring

Femoral vessels

Inguinal ligament

Psoas m.

Superficial inguinal ring

Fossa ovalis

Pubic tubercle

Pectineal m.

Socket for head of femur

Obturator nerve & vessels

Course of spermatic cord and vessels

Figure 11-D

Incidence

Approximately 550 cases have been reported. This hernia tends to occur in elderly, thin, frail women.

Anatomy

The obturator or "adductor" region lies in the lower pelvic area (where it meets the thigh), and extends into the upper third of the thigh. There is a small opening, through which the obturator nerve, artery and vein pass.

Diagnosis

In the vast majority of obturator hernias, the hernia sac contains part of the intestines. In some, because of pressure on the obturator nerve, the patients complain of thigh or knee pain. A discernible mass or lump is rare.

Treatment

The treatment of an obturator hernia is surgical. Occasionally, the hernia is difficult to reduce from within the abdomen, and an incision in the thigh may be needed as well.

Other Hernias of the Pelvic Floor

Other hernias of the pelvis may occur. These are even less common than the other hernias already discussed in this chapter.

Following childbirth, women may develop hernias of the bladder or rectum which protrude into the vagina. These include: urethrocele (prolapse — or downward displacement— of the urethra into the vagina); cystocele (prolapse of the bladder into the vagina); enterocele (prolapse of the superior vagina or peritoneal cavity into the vagina); and rectocele (prolapse of the rectum into the vagina). These hernias are treated surgically by gynecologists.

Internal Hernias

There are many possible defects in the abdomen itself which occasionally occur and trap a loop of intestine. These are usually defects of the membrane which carries the circulation to the intestine (mesentery), a defect of the formation of the mesentery, a defect of a fold in the mesentery, or a defect of the various structures which make up the internal surface of the abdomen. These defects account for approximately one percent of intestinal obstructions.

The repair of unusual internal hernias may be made following typical surgical methods, adapted to the special circumstances of the hernia. Results generally are excellent.

These internal hernias are extremely well documented and illustrated in *Hernia Surgical Technique and Anatomy* by Skandalakis, Gray, Mansberger, Colburn and Skandalakis, 1989.

Summary

The human anatomy is such that hernias in the abdominal cavity occur in a wide variety of locations. The hernias discussed in this chapter are rare, and their symptoms may be elusive. Some physicians never see the more unusual ones in their entire professional career. Identification of these hernias requires a thorough knowledge of the anatomy, an inquisitive mind, and skill in diagnosis.

Chapter Twelve

Preparation for Hernia Surgery

In most cases, hernia repair can be scheduled to the convenience of the patient. In such instances, careful consideration can be given to each facet of the procedure.

Naturally, it is of *great* benefit to diagnose a hernia as early as possible in its development. Most hernias grow progressively worse, and some, such as the incarcerated hernia, can deteriorate quite rapidly.

When *emergency* hernia surgery is necessary, most of the following preparations are completed, but in a more condensed fashion. **The additional risks and inconvenience associated with emergency hernia surgery should not dissuade those suspected of having a hernia from seeking prompt medical attention; hernias do *not* vanish of their own accord.**

The first step of *any* hernia treatment is, of course, to complete a diagnosis by a qualified medical professional. No matter how much you respect a family member, neighbor or friend, unless he or she is a physician, they cannot provide qualified medical judgment. *Never ignore a possible hernia.*

When diagnosis is complete, treatment options should be discussed in detail. This includes the pros and cons of each treatment choice, as well as the risks associated with any "waiting time".

Since most hernias are best treated with surgery, we will describe the *typical* preparations for hernia surgery (either outpatient or hospitalized surgery).

Your Medical History

A complete health/medical history relative to your hernia and any prior illnesses should be taken. This should include:

1. *The time of onset of the hernia* and description of any contributing events. This information is particularly valuable in insurance cases, such as Workman's Compensation.

2. *Previous operations,* including the types of surgery, date of surgery, and a description of associated complications, if any.

3. *The presence of other serious illnesses,* including heart disease, pneumonia, high blood pressure, history of fainting, unusual childhood diseases, or emotional problems. History of previous unusual or prolonged bleeding is extremely important and should be discussed in detail.

4. *Allergies to any medications should be detailed.* Drugs which have caused an allergic reaction should be identified and the nature and extent of the reaction should be described. For example, if the patient has taken penicillin in the past, with subsequent rash or other allergic reaction, then penicillin should not be used. (Many other antibiotics are available and one will be substituted.) Allergic reactions should be

differentiated from functional or nervous reactions, such as that "queasy" feeling we sometimes get when we go to the dentist's or doctor's office. Sometimes the reaction is not one of allergy, but is related to the total dose of the drug used, or to the additives, such as adrenalin, which accompany a local anesthetic. The more detailed the history, the more valuable the information to the surgeon and the anesthesiologist.

5. **Any habits that may influence the outcome of the surgery should be discussed** *honestly* **during the pre-operative evaluation.** Do you smoke? How much? Do you drink alcohol? How much and how often? Do you take Vitamin E and/or aspirin on a daily basis? (These products interfere with platelet activity and may cause bleeding during or after surgery.) Other habits, such as exercise, the use of coffee, tea, colas, etc., should all be discussed with your physician prior to surgery.

Author's Note: General surgeon, Dr. Percy Edgecombe, states: "I found that almost all of my patients would stop smoking when I told them about the pain and complications smokers experience post-operatively. Three weeks made a big difference."

---

6. **Medications you routinely take are extremely important.** You should give the brand or generic name of the drug, the dose in milligrams, and the frequency of intake. All of this information will be listed in your chart and will be available for review by your anesthesiologist and other members of the operating team. After surgery, these medicines may have to be re-ordered, so this information should be exact. *It's a good idea to bring your medicine along with you during your examination.* This way, any necessary information is immediately (and accurately) available.

7. A detailed review of each body system and symptoms should be obtained. You should discuss with your physician any recent weight changes, fatigue or dizziness, or episodes of blindness. You should mention if you have shortness of breath, recurrent cough or sputum (phlegm). This history will help evaluate your lungs. You should discuss symptoms of chest pain or irregular or rapid heart rate. These symptoms will help evaluate your heart. You should describe any indigestion or constipation. (These symptoms help evaluate the hernia and the possibility of a sliding hernia.) You should also tell your physician if you are having any problems with urination, such as frequency, "dribbling", difficulty starting or stopping, or the need to get up to urinate during the night. And, finally, you should discuss any other conditions that you may have, such as arthritis, pain during walking, or episodes of gout.

All of your symptoms paint a general picture of your health and are very helpful in the pre-operative evaluation of your ability to tolerate the surgery.

8. Family history should be discussed. If your hernia is indirect (congenital), other members of the family will often have had hernia surgery. Problems that other blood relatives have had, such as intolerance of general anesthesia, bleeding tendencies (such as hemophilia) should be mentioned. An example is the condition hyperthermia, an extreme febrile (fever) response to general anesthesia. Hyperthermia is a congenital condition, or reaction, to anesthetic agents and may be fatal unless recognized and treated immediately. A family history is the only means of identifying hyperthermia before surgery is performed. If known, the problem is easily avoided.

9. The nature of your work and the physical requirements of your work should be discussed. Your convalescence and post-operative activities can be programmed on the basis of this work and exercise history.

10. **The health of your spouse, live-in or roommate should be discussed.** This is important for two reasons. First, someone should be available to help you the first night of surgery. Second, if your spouse requires medical care and/or lifting by you, arrangements must be made for alternate care of the spouse. As 90% of hernias are being repaired as *outpatient* procedures, it is extremely important to have a healthy companion who is available to help you with your care that first post-operative night.

If your physician knows as much as possible about you, he or she will more capably and efficiently manage your post-operative care. A "good patient" comes to the physician's office prepared to discuss all of the above. *Frequently, it is helpful to make notes prior to the first visit, and to bring your notes with you.*

About the Physical Examination

A physical examination should be performed to carefully evaluate your general health. Your blood pressure should be taken, along with your temperature and pulse. The eyes should be examined. Pinpoint pupils and the pupil reaction should be noted. (Pinpoint pupils are commonly noted and this is often a reminder that the patient is taking eyedrops.) Some eyedrops are so powerful that they can cause a reaction which may keep the patient under anesthetic for 12 hours instead of the planned one hour! Your mouth should be evaluated and the condition of the teeth (or their absence) should be noted. This is particularly important if a general anesthetic is to be used. Your neck should be examined for flexibility and the presence of unusual lumps. Your lungs should be listened to with a stethoscope for signs of bronchitis or other respiratory problems. The heart should be examined for murmurs, irregularities or abnormal sounds. Your abdomen should be felt for the presence of abdominal masses or tenderness, or liver or spleen enlargement. The hernia should be re-examined relative to its size and exact location. The inguinal areas should be examined for hernias and other problems. At this time the male genitalia should be examined and any co-existing condition, such as a hydrocele, should be measured and described. In middle-aged and older male patients, the prostate should be carefully examined. If the patient is over 40, a rectal examination also should be performed. If the patient is female, the urethra should be examined if there are symptoms of obstruction to the urinary flow. Also in the female patient, pelvic examination and pap smears should be updated. Extremities should be checked and any abnormality, skin temperature and color should be noted. Rashes should be evaluated, along with the presence of varicose veins or edema (swelling). Arterial circulation to the feet should be noted. Lastly, you should be examined for enlarged lymph nodes in the neck, armpit or groin. A more comprehensive physical examination should be performed if indicated by the history and clinical condition.

Should Anything More Be Done?

After you have had a complete history and physical, and before the surgery is performed, you should have a routine blood count and urinalysis. The blood count may reveal an unexpected anemia, or an abnormality of the white cells. Urinalysis is also important as it reflects "good health" or may reveal an unexpected problem. If there is any history of heart or lung disease, or if you're 40 or older, you should have a chest x-ray and an electrocardiogram. You should have further laboratory studies according to your need. For example, if you are diabetic, a fasting blood sugar should be obtained. If you have a history of bleeding tendency, a prothrombin time, or partial thromboplastin time (blood clotting factor analysis) should be performed. All of these studies should be "current", i.e., routine laboratory work should be performed within the preceding week and the chest x-ray and EKG within the preceding month.

The pre-operative evaluation should be complete. Remember you are going to be taken through a major surgical procedure. *This is not the time to cut corners.*

Your surgeon should discuss the surgery, its risks, and the alternatives with you in detail. If you have any questions, these should be answered at this time. The staff should then provide directions to the surgical facility. You should also be advised on how to properly prepare yourself for surgery.

You should be told:

- To cancel surgery if you are sick, such as with a cold or upper respiratory infection.

- To have no food or liquid in your stomach for the preceding six hours.

- To take all your usual medications, unless specifically advised otherwise. These medicines should be discussed in detail. All heart medicines should be taken (with just a sip of water). If you take insulin, the proper dosage for the morning of the surgery should be discussed. All medications should be discussed and all of this written down and a copy given to you.

- To make certain your skin is clean, you should be instructed to shower with special soap. To avoid post-operative constipation, you may be advised to take an enema the night or morning before surgery. (This seems like an onerous chore, but it is truly easy if you will use a Fleet's enema, which is specially packaged and easy to use.)

Patients should continue to be physically active while waiting for the surgery. If the hernia can be reduced, or is otherwise comfortable, the patient should enjoy his or her usual physical activities. Hopefully, all of this preparation will allow a pleasant, uneventful operation and post-operative experience.

Summary

To prepare for surgery, patients should give a detailed history and receive a physical examination. This should be accompanied by laboratory analysis and detailed *written* instructions so that they will have the best possible understanding of all the details before, during and after the surgery. A well informed patient is more relaxed during the operation and the post-operative period, and usually has an easier recuperation.

Most of all, remember that the best antidote for fear is information. Have a question? Ask. Afraid you'll forget something? Use a pen and note pad and *write it down!*

Chapter Thirteen

Anesthesia for Hernia Surgery

Introduction

In this chapter, the different types of anesthesia usually used during hernia repair will be discussed. By understanding what is being done to care for you, hopefully you will be reassured, relaxed, and may even find the experience to be enjoyable.

Anesthesia

Anesthesia is a very important part of your overall medical and surgical care, and requires knowledge and cooperation on your part.

Many hernia patients are concerned about the anesthesia they will be given during a hernia repair surgery. Questions about the differences between general, epidural, spinal and local anesthesia are very common. In fact, you *should* ask lots of questions. **The most pressing issues usually are: "Will I have pain during the surgery?" and "What will I do about postoperative discomfort?"**

Please feel free to express any concerns and ask as many questions as you like. Your anesthesiologist is concerned about your comfort and safety.

About Your Anesthesiologist

An anesthesiologist is a physician who, following medical school, has completed several years of additional training in anesthesia and critical care. This physician is an expert member of the surgical team and works closely with the surgeon to provide the best possible care before, during, and after surgery. The anesthesiologist is present continuously throughout your operation. When a physician specially trained in anesthesiology is attending to your needs, the surgeon is able to devote his complete attention to other aspects of the surgery.

About Anesthesia

Anesthesia literally means "without sensation". Modern medicine benefits enormously from the advances made in the field of anesthesiology. A wide variety of anesthetic techniques allows your surgeon to tailor the care to each patient's specific needs.

In all cases, the patients will speak to the anesthesiologist prior to surgery. The patient's medical history, current physical condition, and medicines being taken, will all be discussed and evaluated. Any laboratory work or test made by the patient's medical doctor will also be reviewed.

The anesthetic to be used is determined based on this information, the type and length of surgery, and the needs of the surgeon. Of course, whenever possible, the patient's thoughts and desires will be important factors in the decision-making process. The anesthesiologist will give instructions about preparing for surgery. These preparations are essential in order to provide a safe anesthetic, and must be followed very carefully. Also, at this time, the patient and his or her family will have an opportunity to ask any questions they may have.

Dr. Marc Gipsman recently gave a general anesthesia for one of the author's patients, and he was asked what he specifically discussed during his preoperative interview. Here is his answer:

"I review the history and recent physical as submitted by the surgeon. I check all of the laboratory reports. The values should be within normal limits, and the studies should be appropriate to the patient's health and history. I then talk to the patient relative to any prior problems with anesthetic agents. I am particularly interested in their allergies to medicines, known history of prior anesthetic problems, and their family history of anesthetic problems. I question them about prior cardiopulmonary, hepatic, CNS and renal [heart, lung, liver, brain and nerves, and kidney, respectively] *problems. These are very important, for these organs participate in the acceptance and clearance of the anesthetic agents I will be using. Then I review their wishes relative to the anesthetic techniques.*

"I try to adapt to their wishes or offer a reasonable explanation if their wishes seem inappropriate. I ask about their concerns, such as claustrophobia, teeth or dentures, nausea or vomiting after an anesthetic, and I try to respond.

"Lastly, I perform a physical examination of their airway [jaw, throat, teeth, tongue and neck] *to make certain that they can be intubated* [have a tube passed into the trachea or windpipe] *if needed. I also check the heart for rhythm and*

murmurs, and their lungs to make certain that there has been no change since the preoperative physical examination."

Preparing for Surgery

As mentioned earlier, the patient's knowledge and cooperation are an integral part of successful surgery and recovery. Although each person will receive individualized instructions, the following applies to all surgical patients:

- For out-patient surgery, patients will need to arrange for someone to take them home, as they must not drive for at least 24 hours following surgery.

- The patient will be asked to provide a location and telephone number where he or she can be contacted prior to, and after, surgery.

- For morning surgery, do not eat or drink anything (even water or coffee) for at least eight hours before surgery — this usually means *nothing* to eat or drink after midnight.

- For afternoon surgery, do not eat or drink anything after 7:00 a.m. A *light* breakfast *prior* to 7:00 a.m. MAY be admissible. **This should be discussed in detail with the anesthesiologist.**

- Any regular medications should be discussed with the surgical counselors, who will then pass this information on to the surgical staff. Patients will be told which specific medicines should be taken the morning of surgery.

- Patients should take any heart or blood pressure medication with a small sip of water at their normal time, unless instructed otherwise.

During Surgery

Before the anesthetic is started, monitors will be applied to assess heart rhythm (EKG), blood pressure and oxygen intake continuously during surgery.

For most hernia procedures on adults, the anesthetic involved is called "local, with monitored anesthesia care (MAC)". This ensures that the patient is made absolutely comfortable during all phases of the surgical procedure (including before and after the surgery).

Every patient is unique and, therefore, every anesthetic must be individualized for the maximum safety and effectiveness. Throughout surgery, the anesthesiologist will:

- Deliver the most appropriate anesthetic
- Monitor and manage all vital functions
- Adjust anesthetic level as required
- Provide additional medication if indicated

The anesthesiologist will be with the patient continuously from the moment anesthetic begins until the patient is safely in the care of the recovery-room personnel.

As with *any* medical procedure, there is the possibility of complications from anesthesia. The vast majority of possible problems are minor.

What Is General Anesthesia?

If you are under *general* anesthesia, you will "sleep" during the entire surgery. The anesthesiologist will give combinations of drugs intravenously or as a gas, which you inhale. Some drugs relax your muscles; others introduce sleep; still others decrease perception of pain. All are given in dosages and combinations according to your body, your needs, and the surgeon's requirements. Changes are made continually based on your heart rate, blood pressure, and breathing during surgery. Anesthesiologists today have learned to give microdoses of anesthetics that are ultra fast-acting and able to clear from your body quickly. Therefore, you will awaken very quickly when you arrive in the recovery room.

General anesthesia is most frequently the choice for young children and young adults, but its possible side effects (nausea, and a "hangover") make it the second choice for the mature adult with an uncomplicated inguinal, umbilical, femoral or other small abdominal wall hernia. The author's first choice, local anesthesia with monitored anesthesia care (MAC), will be discussed in the next section.

What Is Local Anesthesia?

Local anesthesia is the injection of local anesthetic agents into the tissue, very similar to what you would receive in the dentist's office. The anesthetic is injected into the field, and into the nerve supply, in the operative area, so that there is complete anesthesia during the operation. Some patients are quite concerned about the needles and about the possibility that they might experience pain. Others, usually older patients, have problems with their heart or lungs and need to be carefully monitored during the operation. Therefore, the anesthesiologist may supplement the local anesthetic with Managed Anesthesia Care (MAC). This gives the best of all worlds for the patients, as they are comfortable and carefully monitored throughout the operation. A combination of local with MAC is extremely safe. More often than not it is used in patients where general anesthetic is contra-indicated.

Describe Local Anesthesia with MAC

Dr. Martin Mann, an anesthesiologist in San Diego, provides MAC to the author's patients on occasion and describes a typical process:

"A nurse will start a flow of sterile fluids through intravenous tubing that is connected to a short plastic tube in a vein in one of your hands or forearms. (This whole set-up is known as an "IV".) These fluids keep your body well hydrated and the "IV" provides a way to give medication during all phases of your surgery. I then meet you (the patient) in the preoperative holding room. I review your medical records, talk to you, and finalize the decision about the type of anesthesia you will receive. If necessary, you will be given Versed® or Valium® via the "IV" to decrease your anxiety; this may also produce amnesia during the surgery. The operating room nurse and I will then push your gurney into the operating room, and we help you move yourself onto the operating table. We make certain that you are comfortable on the table before placing monitors. The monitors include: (1) electrocardiogram (EKG) pads on your chest so that we have a visual display of your heart tracing. (2) a blood pressure cuff placed on one arm to automatically record and display your blood pressure at three-minute intervals, and (3) a pulse oximeter attached to one fingertip with a padded clip. The

oximeter measures the amount of oxygen present in the blood traveling through your finger. If there is enough oxygen in your finger, we know there is enough oxygen everywhere else in your body. Monitoring, using the EKG, blood pressure cuff, and oximeter is continuous throughout the surgery. Also, oxygen is routinely given via small plastic tubes next to your nose. I then give the intravenous anesthesia in small doses until you are just right. I usually use fentanyl, which is similar to morphine, but has a faster onset and shorter duration of action. Sometimes I use Pentothal®, Valium®, or more Versed®."

At this point, the surgeon is allowed to give the local anesthetic. Usually about half an ounce of local anesthetic is injected into the tissues using a small needle to infiltrate the operative site. The surgeon then scrubs up for the operation while the nurse "preps" your skin with a cleansing agent and drapes you with sterile linen. This delay gives the local anesthetic time to work. Dr. Mann continues:

"I sit next to your head and observe you and your monitors. I answer your questions and act as needed to assist you and the operating room personnel. (I even scratch noses on request.) More local anesthesia is given if needed and I continue to provide additional intravenous anesthesia as necessary; this is an on-going process during the surgery. It is extremely unusual for patients to experience any discomfort. However, if necessary, general anesthesia can be given quickly and easily."

The patient often sleeps lightly during the surgery, but he or she can awaken and move about a little on the operating table. Some patients join in the conversation. Others try to entertain us with jokes and witticisms.

Author's note: We enjoy visiting; although, we've heard almost all of the doctor jokes!

During the operation, the surgeon, his or her assistant, and the nurse are very busy identifying structures and handling them carefully, so there is often a quiet, business-like discussion.

After your wound has been sutured and bandaged, you help yourself onto the gurney and the nurse and anesthesiologist take you into the recovery room where you are offered clear liquids.

Author's note: That's a very brief description of local anesthesia with MAC. When local with MAC was first offered, I tried to convince my patients that it was preferable. Now, realizing that most patients enjoy it, I simply state that fact. However, if the patient prefers to be asleep, we schedule the general anesthesia.

What Is Epidural Anesthesia?

Epidural anesthesia is also available. **This is an injection of local anesthetic alongside, but not into, the spinal canal.** Like local anesthetic, epidural anesthesia allows the patient to be free of pain, yet able to move about, cough, and expose the hernia before its repair. Some centers, such as Dr. Lichtenstein's group in Los Angeles, prefer epidural anesthesia for inguinal hernia repair, use it frequently and report that their patients enjoy it. Most of the author's patients are so comfortable with local with MAC, that epidural anesthetic is rarely requested.

What Is Spinal Anesthesia?

Spinal anesthesia eliminates muscle movement and pain sensation in the lower body. **This results from an injection of a small amount of local anesthesia into the spinal canal.** This is an excellent choice for repairing large hernias where relaxation is helpful, and when the hernia is repaired in conjunction with some other surgery, such as a prostatectomy. The patient can be awake or asleep as he or she wishes. In the author's experience, the patient may have trouble urinating immediately following a spinal anesthetic. If the urologist is operating on the prostate, however, then a catheter is left in the bladder and any difficulty voiding is eliminated.

So, Which Anesthesia Is Best?

Most *adult* patients with a routine inguinal, femoral, umbilical, or other small abdominal wall hernia, do exceptionally well when local anesthesia with MAC is used. It has the advantage of rapid recovery of function and fewer side effects. Older patients with major heart or lung illnesses also seem to tolerate local with MAC exceptionally well. In fact, this anesthetic is often *the safest* for older patients with heart or lung disease.

If the patient is young or "squeamish", it's okay to ask for general anesthesia — the surgeons and anesthesiologists will work with the patient to assure comfort *and* surgical success!

Following Surgery

The anesthesiologist and specially trained nurses will make the short recovery period as pleasant as possible. Medications to lessen discomfort can be administered if needed. In most cases, the anesthesiologist will visit prior to the patient's release in order to evaluate recovery and answer any questions. The patient and the person taking them home will receive post-operative instructions from the post-operative nurse.

Most importantly, patients must not drive a car, operate any type of machinery (including a sewing machine) or make any important decisions for at least 24 hours following surgery. (If additional medications are prescribed for pain, a longer period of time may be required.) Remember, all surgery results in disturbances of the body's natural routine and requires a reasonable time for recovery. It is recommended that the patient rest quietly for the remainder of the surgical day. Post-operative tiredness is normal and can last up to a week. The surgeon should be contacted with any special concerns.

Types of Anesthetic

GENERAL ANESTHESIA — Complete unconsciousness without any sensation or awareness of surroundings or passage of time. Requires a breathing tube.

REGIONAL ANESTHESIA — Usually administered along with a sedative, regional anesthesia is injected around a group of nerves in order to numb the surgical area.

LOCAL ANESTHESIA — Often given along with a sedative, local anesthesia is applied directly to the area of surgery and does not itself directly effect overall consciousness.

EPIDURAL ANESTHESIA — Local anesthetic injected alongside the spinal canal. Provides complete numbness to the lower body, but patient remains conscious.

SPINAL ANESTHESIA — Local anesthesia is injected into the spinal canal. The resulting lack of feeling and *muscle relaxation* may be helpful during some procedures.

MANAGED ANESTHETIC CARE ("MAC") — Allows the minimum amount of anesthetic to be administered with the security of additional anesthetic immediately available, if needed. This protects the patient and minimizes anesthetic side effects.

Chapter Fourteen

"We need to realize and to affirm anew that nursing is one of the most difficult arts. Compassion may provide the motive, but knowledge is our only working power."

M. Adelaide Nutting

Nursing Care

Nurses make their presence known throughout medical care today, and hernia care is no exception. Nurses have established themselves as the backbone of patient care. They staff our hospitals 24 hours a day, seven days a week. Trauma nurses fly on helicopters, arrive at the scene and perform resuscitative procedures. Intensive care nurses provide invaluable constant bedside nursing, performing functions normally performed by interns at some institutions. Surgical nurses assist at heart surgery, operate the heart-lung machine, and are an invaluable part of the surgical team. Some have expanded their role to be operating room supervisors, or they specialize and are replacing physicians and administrators at many levels of care.

Nurses are the nucleus of the staff in out-patient surgical centers, providing recovery room management, as well as taking the responsibility for instruments, supplies, and sterility. House calls, no longer a routine for physicians, are now provided by nurses. With training, the nurses are thoroughly conversant with the problems of medical and surgical patients alike. They have the patience to visit and care for, to gently assist, to answer questions, and to reassure.

Wherever your hernia is cared for, nurses will be there. They will help create a safe and comfortable environment for you.

Historical Review

Nursing has been described as one of the oldest arts, and yet one of the youngest professions. Some people believe the profession began with Florence Nightingale; but, the *"act"* of nursing and giving care is as old as mankind. For primitive man, the nurse was often a slave and, later, she was a domestic.

The pronoun *"she"* is appropriate and is commonly used when discussing nurses, because the profession is so related to the evolving roles of women in society. The word *"nurse"* has its roots with the Latin word *"nutrix"* which means *"nursing mother"*. However, the nursing ranks today include men, and they are equally effective and nurturing.

As medical knowledge evolved, it became obvious that *"nurturing"* alone would not cure illness. The development of nursing over time parallels scientific developments.

Perhaps no person or event exemplifies this evolution better than Florence Nightingale.

The Nightingale Revolution

Florence Nightingale (1820-1910) was named after the city of her birth, Florence, Italy. Nightingale's parents were traveling on the Continent at the time of her birth. She was educated in literature, philosophy, religion, science, and higher mathematics and, by the time she was 17, spoke two foreign languages; she was probably better educated than most men of her time. At a very early age, she expressed a desire to enter nursing, but she was not encouraged by her parents. At the age of 27, she enrolled in a program for nursing at Kaiserwerth, Germany. Later she studied in Paris under the Sisters of Charity. Returning to London, she assumed an administrative position as superintendent of The Establishment for Gentlewomen During Illness. In her year there, she created a model institution by the standards of the day.

In 1854, Great Britain was engaged in the Crimean War. Wounded soldiers were cared for at a base in Scutari, where, without nursing care, the mortality rate was high. Following extremely critical publicity in the British newspaper, the Secretary of War, Sir Sidney Herbert, defied precedence and invited Florence Nightingale to take a contingent of nurses to Scutari and help treat the wounded. Nightingale accepted the challenge and went to Scutari with 32 nurses. She introduced sanitary science through female nursing in Scutari and reduced the death rate of the wounded from 42% to 2% (1854-1855).

She wrote extensively during the next five years, describing the frightful, but preventable, mortality of the war. She showed the value of sanitary science in medical care. She wrote an authoritative text on modern nursing and established The Army Medical School at Fort Pitt, Chatham. She chose its faculty and founded the first training school for nurses at St. Thomas Hospital in 1860. Florence Nightingale was truly a remarkable woman. She was educated, dedicated, capable of writing and leading.

Florence Nightingale was admired for her devotion to her patients. She often visited the sickest patients in the evening, following a long day of administrative duties, accompanied only by her "lamp", a candle holder with a wind shield which prevented the flame from being extinguished. The grateful survivors of Scutari dubbed her, *"The lady with the lamp"*.

Florence Nightingale was truly ahead of her time. Many of her contributions to sanitary science preceded those of Semmelweis, Lister and Pasteur.

Today, advances in nursing education have created professional nurses whose capabilities are unlimited.

Chapter Fifteen

Post-Operative Care

Today's emphasis on *out-patient* hernia surgery has many advantages over hospitalization: most people prefer to recuperate in familiar surroundings; costs associated with hospitalization are eliminated; and hospital beds and staffing can be utilized for more urgent cases.

And today's hernia patients usually are "cheated" out of complaints about the hospital food, "slow" responses to urgent requests for attention, and uncomfortable beds.

Instead, adult hernia patients most often return to their homes, with family members or friends providing gentle support. Not only do modern sophisticated surgical techniques greatly reduce the trauma of hernia surgery, but anesthetics and pain medications used today significantly reduce any discomfort. Highly-skilled visiting nurses effectively monitor each patient's progress. All these advances provide hernia surgery patients with far more comfortable post-operative recovery, in less time and with fewer disruptions to their normal routine. And, many patients find that their convalescence often seems to draw family members and friends closer through the shared experience.

Recovery following a hernia repair is usually rapid and the patient remains fairly comfortable. There may be some incision discomfort, but this should not prevent the patient from getting up and about. As soon as healing allows, patients should be active, but not to the point of fatigue. Patients are encouraged to return to normal activities as soon as they feel well enough. Even exercise such as walking, running and swimming is encouraged.

For the first few weeks, however, heavy lifting and competitive sports should be avoided. Patients who are generally active seem to heal more quickly, and experience fewer complications. Those patients who maintain a sensible exercise program before surgery, seem to benefit.

Medications You Should have Available

Prior to non-emergency surgery, patients should make a careful inventory of any prescriptions and over-the-counter medications used on a regular basis.

Be certain that any *prescriptions* are up-to-date and on hand. Patients generally resume taking daily medications (such as high blood pressure, thyroid, etc.) immediately following surgery.

In addition, prior to having surgery, patients should make certain that the following over-the-counter products are available:

1. *Tylenol®*. Tylenol® is very helpful for incision pain. The usual adult dose is two tablets every four hours. It is particularly valuable because it usually doesn't cause stomach upset.

2. **Other medications such as *Ibuprofen* (Motrin®), Advil®, or Nuprin®.** These medications are extremely helpful when the incision is a little swollen or sore, although they *may* cause stomach upset.

3. ***Liquid antacids* should be in the house and available for use.** If the patient is prone to indigestion, additional prescriptive medicine, such as Tagamet®, Zantac®, or Pepcid® should be obtained. If these are occasionally taken by the patient on a regular basis, any prescriptions should be refilled and immediately available.

4. ***Stool softeners* are extremely valuable in the post-operative period, because pain medications tend to constipate.** Taking a stool softener allows the moisture to be retained in the stool, so that constipation will not occur. These are available over the counter. Look for the adult dose, 240mg. daily of Surfak®, Colace® or the generic, Docusate Sodium.

5. ***Any other medicines* that might be valuable to *you*.** For instance, surgery *may* cause a flair-up of gout, and therefore, if you've had gout in the past, your gout medication should be available. (In fact, it is better to start taking gout medicine prior to surgery and stay on it during your first post-operative week.)

It is wise to think about your health in response to stress. If you tend to have a problem with bodily functions when stressed, be prepared to deal with it. Have the appropriate medications on hand.

6. *A pain medication will be prescribed* **after the operation.** This will be something like Tylenol with codeine®, Vicodin®, Tylox®, or Darvocet-N®, according to your needs and tolerances.

After Release

After release from the out-patient surgery facility (usually about one to two hours after surgery), patients are taken directly home, to a local hotel, or to a special convalescent center.

Most surgeons feel that it is important that the patient remain near the locale of the surgery the first night following the operation. In the highly unlikely event of a complication requiring medical treatment, time can be important. Also, this makes the nurse's visit (and physician's, in some cases) much more convenient.

Post-Operative Nursing Visit

A nurse will visit the patient approximately six hours after surgery. This specially-trained medical professional will check temperature and pulse, change the dressing and examine the incision, and will assist with general nursing care.

The nurse also gives instruction in the proper way to get in and out of bed, and confirms that recovery is progressing as it should.

Since most local anesthetics will lose their effectiveness at about this time, the nurse may provide additional pain relief.

Following the nursing visit, most patients go to sleep and begin a comfortable night's rest.

Note: Local drug stores usually close by 9:00 p.m. It is important that any medication needs or changes be evaluated earlier in the evening, while a pharmacist is still available.

Physical Activities the First Day or Two

You should be given an ice bag as you start to recover. This should be left in place for at least four hours. However, you will be asked to also stand and walk about briefly, hourly, the first day, until your normal bed time. You may put the ice bag to one side, during the "stroll".

During the first few days (the first night in particular), *men* are encouraged to wear jockey shorts, or to very simply elevate their scrotum by placing a bathtowel across the thighs when they are lying on their back. The scrotum is placed on the bathtowel and this elevation lessens the swelling of the scrotal contents which so commonly follows any surgery in the groin.

After surgery, patients will want to get in and out of bed without using the abdominal muscles. Performance of a "sit-up" is usually painful at first and should be avoided. Instead, the patient should roll over onto one side or the other, then use his or her arms against the bed to push the upper body into an upright position.

Swelling of the surgical incision post-operatively seems to be universal and is often of considerable concern to the patient. By applying ice to the incision for the first four to eight hours, the swelling is lessened. After the first 24 hours, an application of heat may give some relief to the discomfort and swelling.

Walking and standing are encouraged. However, if you are uncomfortable, it is best to lie down. For many reasons, *sitting*, particularly for long periods of time, does not seem beneficial. After sitting for prolonged periods, it is very difficult to stand and straighten up. Also, there is a tendency for blood to pool in the lower extremities when sitting and this may cause blood clots, particularly for those who have varicose veins.

In general, patients who are active are usually more comfortable and heal more quickly than inactive patients.

Physical Activities the First Week After Surgery

After a routine inguinal hernia repair, it is usually beneficial to be physically active very early in convalescence and to place minimal restrictions on lifting, etc. It seems reasonable to talk about this in terms of sports, because many patients are involved in some sort of physical activity outside of work and are anxious to return to these activities.

Patients should be allowed to start walking just as soon as they feel like it. Walking is encouraged for it helps maintain muscle tone and stimulates the heart and lungs. Patients may be allowed to walk vigorously as soon as they feel like it, starting with the day after surgery. Similarly, jogging is good exercise. Most patients who are active runners start jogging within a few days.

Swimming is also an excellent exercise, and should not in any way stress the *routine* groin hernia repair. However, diving is another matter and should not be attempted in the first few weeks. Patients are encouraged to participate in swimming activities when the sutures or clips have been removed, approximately one week from the surgery.

Other physical exercises, such as stretching and aerobics, should be entered into as soon as the patient feels like it. The patient may participate in these activities in the first week, certainly *not later* than the second week. Some patients maintain an active physical activity program, but stop the program for a few weeks immediately following surgery. If there is a concurrent condition, such as a back problem, it is important to return to a regular exercise program which includes stretching and bending, as soon as possible. Most patients are often cautious and restrict themselves moderately during the first week or two after surgery. Some of this self-imposed restriction is probably in response to the old-fashioned notion that an inguinal hernia patient must have six weeks time off. New techniques do not require this restriction.

Physical Activities After the First Week

Patients generally have concerns about returning to certain sports that they enjoy, such as golf. A golfer should return to the golf course in the first week (carrying his putter and five iron) and, after a few rounds, should very quickly convert to the nine iron, then the seven, and, after a week or so, start to use his or her long irons, then the woods. Golfers often report that a hernia repair helps their game, for they stop swinging so wildly, and hit a straighter ball!

Tennis players are encouraged to return to the courts after a couple of weeks. It is recommend that they play non-competitively for a week or so. Racquetball is very similar. Patients may get onto the court as soon as they want to, but they should avoid throwing themselves against one another or onto the floor, trying to make every shot. Bowling and weightlifting are more demanding and patients are advised to avoid these activities for about three weeks, and then to perform them modestly at first.

Patients want to know how soon they can resume climbing stairs. The usual answer is, "On the way home from the surgery center." When can they start driving a car? "Just as soon as they are off narcotics and their head feels clear." When can they go shopping? Again, "As soon as the head is clear. " What about sexual activities? And the answer is, "As soon as it feels good."

All of these physical activities are put into perspective by simple acts such as coughing or sneezing, acts which usually cannot be avoided and are frequently experienced very early in the post-operative course. These are natural functions, they do occur, and the modern hernia repair resists breakdown in the face of these activities. Similarly, simple acts, such as sports activities or driving the car, prove to be quite safe and reasonable.

Post-Operative Exercises

A graduated exercise program is important for all of us. Good muscle tone is particularly important for maintenance of the integrity of the abdominal wall.

Most patients are anxious to know what sort of activities or exercise they can perform after a hernia repair.

They are also interested to know what exercises they *should* maintain, so they will not develop a recurrence. According to Ruth Fabian, a registered nurse and a registered and licensed physical therapist, the following suggestions are recommended to speed recovery and maintain optimal results:

"The patient can start this program on the day of surgery. The starting position for all of the exercises is lying on the back, on the bed or floor, with no pillows under the head. Flex knees and hips with feet flat on the surface and spaced apart the width of the hips. The relax phase is a return to the starting position." See figure 15-A.

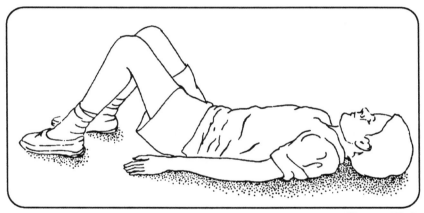

Figure 15-A

"All exercises are to be done three times daily and in repetitions of five, with the position held for a slow count of five. Counting aloud prevents holding one's breath during the hold period."

DAYS ONE THROUGH FIVE

Exercise #1 Ruth continues, "*Raise your head as though looking at something down between the feet. Hold for a count of five. Relax. Repeat to a total of five.*"

Exercise #2 "*Raise your right arm and reach across the body, over and above the left hip. Hold for a count of five. Relax. Raise your left arm and reach across the body for a count of five. Relax. Repeat to a total of five, alternating right and left.*"

"*Now, repeat this series another five times, thus doing a total of ten repetitions of each motion.*"

DAYS SIX THROUGH TEN

"*Note that each motion increases slightly in range. Same start position.*"

Exercise #1 "*Raise your head*", Ruth continues, "*looking toward the feet and raise arms to knee height. Hold for a count of five, counting aloud. Relax. Repeat to a total of five.*"

Exercise #2 "*Raise your right arm and head, reaching across the body, above the left hip. Notice your right shoulder will rise slightly from surface. Hold for a count of five. Relax. Raise your left arm and head, reaching across body to over the right hip. Now the left shoulder rises slightly. Hold, count to five. Relax. Repeat five times. Now repeat these each five times to a total of ten repetitions, remembering the side reaches are to be alternated.*"

DAYS ELEVEN THROUGH FIFTEEN

Exercise #1 *"From the starting position",*Ruth continues, *"raise your arms, head and shoulders until the hands are just above the knees. Hold for a count of five. Relax. Repeat for a total of five."* See figure 15-B.

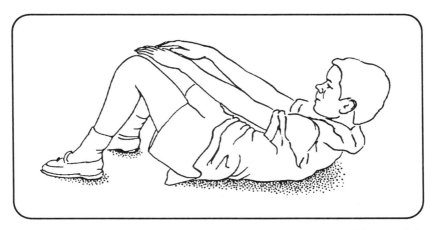

Figure 15-B

Exercise #2 *"Keeping both knees up, raise your right arm and reach across the body above the left hip, raising head and shoulder. Hold for a count of five, relax. Do this using your left arm reaching across. Repeat this exercise, alternating right and left, for a total of five."*

Exercise #3 *"Lower your right leg to surface, keeping left knee bent and right knee straight, and raise the right leg to the height of your left knee. Hold for a count of five. Repeat this right leg raise for a total of five times. Repeat this exercise with the left leg. Do not alternate one-for-one in this exercise.*

"Repeat these exercises, in this order, five times each for a total of ten motions in the exercise period."

After this, you may proceed with single leg raising for a week, double leg raising for the week, and then start sit-ups.

These exercises are very simple, yet they do use the abdominal muscles which are important in the strength of a hernia repair. Because they are gradually introduced, there is no reason to feel that there will be any damage to the hernia repair.

Post-Operative Pain

The pain patients experience is extremely variable. Everyone has their own individual threshold for pain and their own perception of it. It is also important to realize that some patients require considerably more surgery to allow repair of the hernia; others, considerably less.

The type of anesthetic agent seems important, for studies have shown that local anesthesia results in much less post-operative discomfort. In 1990, anesthesiologist, Mark Tverskoy, M.D., Ph.D., published an analysis of post-operative pain after inguinal hernia repairs. He studied patients who had had three types of anesthetic: a general anesthetic, a spinal anesthetic, and those with local and anesthesia supplements, comparable to MAC (Managed Anesthetic Care). He demonstrated that patients had *one-fourth* the post-operative pain when local anesthesia was used. He studied the patients at 24 hours, 48 hours, and again at 10 days. There was a wide variation in the pain perception at 24 and 48 hours, but all the patients seemed to have little discomfort at ten days.

Post-Operative Swelling

Surgical incisions tend to swell during the immediate post-operative period and this swelling is a source of concern to most patients. **This concern is very reasonable, for the patient has just come in with a bulge that needs repair, and the post-operative swelling,** *to the patient,* **is similar to that bulge!** A groin incision seems to swell more than others, possibly because of its location. *This swelling should not be a cause for alarm.* It will revert to normal in a matter of days. The swelling will probably improve more quickly with the application of gentle heat (*after the first twenty-four hours*) and the ingestion of anti-inflamatory medication such as Ibuprofen or Advil®.

Return to Work

If the patient is self-employed or otherwise highly motivated, he or she will probably return to work in the first week, or no later than the second week. Naturally, he or she will not perform unrestricted lifting and physical activity the first week, but can return to the work place, and participate in most of the required physical activities. Patients should be cautioned not to become too tired the first week or two after surgery. They may find their resistance is low and they may be more subject to contracting a cold or the flu. A good plan is to be active for three or four hours, then rest until feeling good again.

Patients who are doing *heavy* physical labor usually return to work in three or four weeks. After a normal convalescence, of about two weeks, a hernia repair will be quite strong and patients should be able to perform active physical labor without risk. When some patients experience pain at the site of the incision, they immediately protect themselves by not performing that physical act again (This is not necessary). Discussing this ahead of time helps the patient gain perspective and understanding.

Many employers are willing to take the patient back to work early in the post-operative period, and will offer modified work requirements.

Questions Commonly Asked

Patients, in spite of the volume of material available to them, still have many questions. Here are some of the most common:

When can I drive?

As soon as you are comfortable. However, you should *not* drive when taking pain medications or sedatives. And remember, don't lift the garage door during the first week.

When can I have a bowel movement?

If you don't have one the first or second day after surgery, don't worry. Do take a stool softener daily. If you don't have a bowel movement the third day after surgery, take your favorite remedy for constipation. Common suggestions are: Milk of Magnesia, a dish of prunes, a suppository, or a Fleets® enema. Whatever works for you is fine.

When may I shower?

When the dressing has been removed. You may remove the dressing yourself on the second day after surgery. A good way to do this is to get into the shower and let the dressing get soaked for a few minutes. Then it will be less likely to adhere to the wound when you remove it.

When are the sutures removed?

Usually on the third to seventh day after surgery. It is preferable not to leave them in beyond the seventh day, as they may begin to cause superficial irritation.

Will the incision hold together if the sutures are removed early?

Yes. An extremely adhesive liquid, called Mastisol®, is applied to the skin, followed by sterile strips to hold the incision together. These Steri-Strips® will stay in place for at least one week, if you are careful with them and do not take prolonged showers or baths.

How long should these Steri-Strips® stay on?

At least seven days from the surgery date.

Do I *have* to take the pain pills?

No. These are simply to help you so that you may be physically active. However, if you are *not* taking pain pills, and are *not* comfortable, you *should* try something. Take two Tylenol®, aspirin, or Advil®, and take them at least four times a day. *There is no need to suffer*.

How long should I use an ice bag?

For at least four hours, and up to 24 hours, if you wish. Take all of the air out of the ice bag. Air doesn't conduct the cold well. Some innovative patients have used a bag of frozen peas instead of ice. After 24 hours, you may try gentle heat at this point and see if it makes you more comfortable.

How do I apply heat?

Use a heating pad, set at **low**, only!

What if I have indigestion?

Take a liquid antacid. Liquid antacids are more effective than tablets. In fact, it is best to have medication for indigestion available in the medicine cabinet before surgery.

What if I have gas?

Take Mylicon-80®, GAS-X®, or a similar "gas" pill. These products can be obtained at your drug store, over the counter. (Some antacids have the anti-gas factor, simethicone, included.)

Why does my incision seem swollen?

It's not uncommon to have some swelling after any operation. The incision and repair produce edema (swelling). In addition, the solutions used to sterilize your skin before the surgery can be irritating, and there may be a slight swelling of the skin wherever the solution was applied. Swelling at the incision may be the width of a finger and still be normal. The swelling of the skin from the prep solutions is usually a soft thickening of the skin and that also is normal. Both of these swellings will gradually disappear with time. If an incision is infected it will be red and warm. If you have any doubts regarding an infected incision, you should see your physician within 24 hours.

If there is swelling of the incision, has the hernia returned?

No.

Is the swelling from the mesh, or patch?

No. When mesh is used, it is *at least* three layers deep in the incision. It does not cause any perceptible swelling.

Why is mesh used?

To allow the repair to be solid and without tension.

What if the testicle is swollen?

If you had a groin hernia, the swelling seen is usually skin swelling from the prep solutions. Sometimes patients mistake this for a swollen testicle. Stop a minute and gently feel the area.. The testicle and cord structures should be soft and approximately the same size as the opposite side. If the testicle is swollen and hard, you should be seen immediately.

What if I have some pain?

It is not uncommon to have pain in a hernia incision. There are nerves which travel through the incision and the suturing may have put pressure on them. This usually stops in a week or so. It is also important to remember that there are three abdominal wall muscles in the groin. These muscles tend to move in separate directions. Following hernia repair in this area, the muscles may adhere to one another briefly and re-institution of movement may cause some pain. This is quite normal.

Summary

Hernia surgery need not be a traumatic experience. Recovering in the comfort of one's home, the *well-prepared* patient will usually have few, if any problems.

Some preparation for the post-operative period is necessary. Friends or relatives should be available for general assistance. Medications and other items of comfort should be purchased prior to surgery and available in the home. A visiting nurse provides further support to the patient and the family, and can also provide additional pain-reducing medication, if necessary. The physician should always be immediately available.

Patients are often fearful of being active in the first few days following hernia repair. However, an active patient usually heals more rapidly and there are several exercises the patient can perform to assist the healing process.

Patients often have questions following surgery and these should be answered. There is no such thing as a stupid question! If the questions addressed in this chapter do not answer all of your concerns, be sure to ask your doctor!

Chapter Sixteen

History of Hernia Surgery

Introduction

All of us have heroes. Some of us are fortunate enough to have been close to men or women who stood above the crowd with their dedication, ability, and love of their profession. Such a man was Dr. H. Glenn Bell, a kindly, unpretentious surgeon who was the Professor of Surgery, during my surgical residency training at the University of California at San Francisco.

Glenn was born on a farm near Hillsboro, Ohio. While a high school student, he worked for a family doctor in the community, helping with care of the doctor's horses and livery. At Glenn's home, a sow had a litter of pigs and some of these piglets had congenital inguinal hernias. Glenn repaired the hernias in the piglets, under the supervision of the family doctor. A surgeon was born.

He received his M.D. degree from the University of Cincinnati at the age of 28, and remained there as intern, resident and then chief resident in general surgery. He then went to the University of California at San Francisco and, one year later, was appointed Chief of the Division of General Surgery in July, 1930.

Glenn's surgical professor in Cincinnati was trained by William Halsted, and Glenn carried on with the meticulous technique characteristic of the Halstedian school. The operative field was always clean and dry. The operation always proceeded with precision.

Glenn was a master of surgical skills. But Glenn was more than a master surgeon. Always gentle with his patients, he understood their problems, and calmed their fears as he took them through a surgical procedure. Glenn led by example. He felt that each surgical resident would represent the quality of the work and training at the University of California at San Francisco.

Glenn was very industrious. After each operation, he would visit with the patient's family, then dictate the procedure, while the resident wrote the post-operative orders. He then returned to the operating room and helped prepare for his next patient. It was not unusual for him to pick up a mop and clean the floor! We very quickly learned not to leave this task undone.

Every Sunday morning, 30 to 40 medical students, interns, and residents would "make rounds" with Glenn. We would present our surgical patients and attempt to gain his approval of our care and results.

Although it was not "fashionable" at the time, Glenn enjoyed using local anesthesia for surgery, and would often perform hernia repairs, under local, on his private patients. One day he removed a thyroid tumor under local anesthesia. It proceeded very smoothly and he conversed with the patient as we operated. As we left the room, he finally said to me, "Do you know why I did that?"

"No", I responded.

"So you'll know how", Glenn replied, "if you ever have to do neck surgery and you don't have an anesthesiologist or general anesthesia available."

Glenn spoke "harshly" to me just once. Three of us were helping him operate on a small baby with a difficult surgical problem. We were deep in the baby's pelvis; eight hands shared a very limited space. I was his resident and was directing the assistants. He prepared for the placement of the first suture of the repair and said, "Don't anybody move". I shifted slightly and improved his exposure. The operation proceeded without a hitch. As we walked out of the operating room, Glenn quietly said, "I know you made it better when you moved, but when I say hold still, hold still."

Glenn was universally loved by his residents. He was also appreciated by the University. In 1961, the University of Cincinnati awarded him an honorary Doctor of Science degree. That same year, the University of California at San Francisco awarded him an honorary Doctor of Law degree.

The history of medicine and surgery is all about our past experiences, our teachers, the people who have gone ahead of us, and have left a legacy, so we can be better physicians and surgeons for our patients.

This chapter is dedicated to H. Glenn Bell, Senior.

Introduction to History of Hernia Surgery

Surgery for the treatment of hernias has come a long way. Major contributors, in addition to surgeons with a particular interest in hernia repair, have been the anatomists, anesthesiologists, and individuals such as Pasteur, Lister and Semmelweis.

Hernias were first mentioned on papyrus documents in Egypt 3,500 years ago, describing the use of snugly fitting bandages for reduction and support of enlarging hernias. These "trusses" were recommended to bind the area to prevent protrusion and "hopefully" eliminate incarceration and gangrene. Medicine had little to offer.

Anatomists

Religious mores forbid the dissection of human bodies until the late middle ages. Before that time, training relied on dissection of animals, such as pigs or sheep, with the assumption that the anatomy of humans was somewhat similar.

With time, dissection of the human body was allowed and the groin began to be defined.

Outstanding individual contributions include:

Adrian Van der Spieghle (1578 -1625). Van der Spieghle held the chair of Anatomy and Surgery at the University of Padua. He first described the lateral margin of the rectus muscles, where the transverse muscle converts from muscle to fascia. Anatomists converted Dr Spieghle's name to the Latin form and referred to the *linea spigelli*. Subsequently, any hernia which developed in this line was labeled a Spigel's, or spigelian hernia.

Antonio De Gimbernat (1734 - 1818). De Gimbernat held the chair of anatomy in Barcelona. He described the ligament later given his name, and advised cutting it to enlarge the femoral ring in the case of incarceration.

Franz K. Hesselbach (1759 - 1816). This German surgeon described the groin, and particularly the posterior (back) wall of the inguinal canal. This area is now called Hesselbach's triangle and is the area where direct inguinal hernias are found.

Astley Pastor Cooper (1768 - 1841). Cooper was both a surgeon and a renowned anatomist. He described the ligament later given his name, as well as other components of the inguinal anatomy, particularly the transversalis fascia.

History of Treatment of Infections

Ignaz Philipp Semmelweis (1818-1865), was a Professor of Obstetrics and pioneered in antisepsis in obstetrics. He was disturbed by the many deaths among women, following childbirth, at the University of Vienna. In his first month in the department, 36 of the newly delivered women died, out of a total of 208. The midwives, operating separately from the physicians, enjoyed a superior success rate. Semmelweis made the astute observation that his students often cared for the obstetrical patients after they had attended morning pathology and morgue rounds. The post mortem room and pathology work, and the subsequent deaths of the mothers, seemed to be related. The midwives, who enjoyed a much more favorable mortality rate, never came to the morgue!

In 1847, a friend and colleague of Semmelweis' died from septicemia after wounding himself with a scalpel during an autopsy. Semmelweis attended his colleague's post mortem and noted that the lesion in his colleague's body was similar to the kind observed in the obstetric ward in women with puerpural fever (an infection after childbirth). Semmelweis deduced that it was the scalpel that had transferred the "invisible poison" from the corpse to the unfortunate physician.

Convinced that the infection was transmitted in this way, Semmelweis issued stringent orders; before visiting a patient, everyone was to wash their hands carefully and the wards were to be cleansed with calcium chloride. After these precautions were instituted, the mortality rate from puerpural fever in the ward fell rapidly from 12% to almost zero.

Unfortunately, when published, Semmelweis' work was not well presented. His contemporaries viewed his work as controversial and gave it a poor reception. Not long thereafter, Semmelweis, suffering from organic brain disease and dementia, was institutionalized, and died. Semmelweis' illness and mental deterioration may explain his failure to properly present his facts.

Louis Pasteur (1822-1895), was a French chemist and the founder of the science of bacteriology. His studies of wine fermentation led to the discovery that destruction of germs by heat preserved wine. Furthermore, Pasteur demonstrated that microorganisms, found all around us, were the cause of infection and decay. Pasteur developed an aseptic approach which was later converted to medical use. The milk that we drink today is "pasteurized" by the use of heat to kill bacteria. Our operating rooms use heat to sterilize most of the surgical instruments.

Joseph Lister (1827-1912), was an English Quaker and Professor of Surgery at Glasgow. He learned of the effectiveness of carbolic acid as a disinfectant for sewage. Lister then selected carbolic acid for use as an antiseptic in both the prevention and treatment of infections in surgical wounds. In addition to the "antiseptic dressings", a carbolic spray was designed for use in the operating room. Lister's patients enjoyed a greatly improved success rate. In 1867 he published the manuscript "On the Antiseptic Principle in the Practice of Surgery". His work was immediately embraced in Europe and America, but was not generally accepted in Great Britain for nearly 25 years. When Pasteur's ideas were popularized, Lister adapted his techniques to incorporate Pasteur's concept of asepsis.

The Discovery of Penicillin

It is easy to forget that the discovery of antibiotics and their use in the treatment of infection is a 20th Century event. **Arthur Fleming** (1881- 1955), was a Scottish scientist working in a modest laboratory in 1928, when he made this remarkable discovery! Fleming noted mold growing around one of his petri dishes containing a culture of staphylococcus aureus ("staph"), which was being grown for analysis. It is thought that the mold grew from scraps of food left by Fleming's co-workers.

The "staph" bacteria grew throughout the petri dish, except in the area immediately around the mold. The mold seemed to destroy the "staph". Through the study of this phenomenon, penicillin, our first antibiotic, was developed.

Today, we have a seemingly unlimited number of different antibiotics available to us. "Medical Letter", in May, 1990, enumerated 48 different antibiotics and their clinical indications.

Treatment of infections in surgery now include all the principles of asepsis, coupled with the use of antibiotic agents to prevent infections.

History of Anesthesia

In the 1800's, surgeons used speed to limit their patients' agony during operations. In 1824 Henry Hill Hickman (1800-1830) published a work in which he described the successful use of carbon dioxide (CO_2) on animals during surgery. In 1818 Faraday discovered ether, and later went on to pioneer in electricity.

Crawford Long (1815-1878), a modest practitioner in Jefferson, Georgia was the first to use ether on humans. In 1842 the administration of ether to James Venable was recorded in his log with *"removal of tumour - $2.00"*. In 1878 he published his experiences with the repeated use of ether anesthesia.

William Thomas Green Morton (1819-1868), a dentist and medical student, while enrolled in Harvard Medical School, gave ether anesthesia to a patient in October, 1846 to allow excision of a tumor of the neck. Dr. Morton had obtained experience giving ether to dogs for tooth extractions. Dr. John Collins Warren, Chief Surgeon at the Massachusetts General Hospital, performed the operation and was so impressed by the anesthetic, that he turned to his audience and said, *"Gentlemen, this is no humbug"*. Because Crawford Long failed to publish his use of ether until two years later, Thomas Morton was given credit for the first use of ether anesthesia.

The "Ether Dome" at Massachusetts General Hospital has been preserved as a national monument, enshrining Dr. Morton's demonstration of the value of ether. Incidentally, this is the smallest national park.

Subsequently, multiple inhalation anesthetic agents, such as chloroform and cyclopropane, were introduced, refined, and replaced. Far superior general anesthetic agents have been developed and are currently being used.

Ether anesthesia, because of its flammable characteristics, is no longer used. Today in fact, ether cannot be found within the hospital.

History of Local Anesthesia

The first local anesthetic discovered was cocaine. Natives in the Andes Mountains of South America chewed the leaves of the coca bush for its mind altering effect. Extracted in the laboratory the substance, cocaine, was found to produce numbness when applied to the tongue. Injections into tissue produced local anesthesia.

Local anesthesia was used by the Austrian Karl Koller (1857-1944) in 1884. In 1898, August Karl Gustav Bier (1861-1949) demonstrated analgesia of the lower extremities by injecting cocaine into the spinal canal. Bier, a surgeon was so interested in developing spinal anesthesia, that he volunteered to allow the first spinal to be given to himself. The needle did not fit the syringe, and there was a great loss of his spinal fluid during the procedure. He had a spinal headache for nine days.

Procaine (Novocaine) was synthesized by Ineharn in 1904, and was used for spinal anesthesia in 1905. Subsequent local anesthetics have been developed and refined. Safer and more stable local anesthetic agents, with a prolonged duration of activity and lower levels of toxicity, were subsequently developed. Lidocaine (Xylocaine®) was synthesized in 1943 and clinically introduced in 1947. Subsequently Carbocaine® and Marcaine® were introduced. These agents now allow safe administration of local anesthesia.

History of Hernia Surgeons

The Italian surgeon, **Edoardo Bassini,** M.D. (1844-1924), is known as the father of hernia surgery. He published results of a series of 227 operations performed between 1884 and 1889 with an incidence of recurrence of under 10%, and only one death. This astounded his contemporaries , for they were experiencing a 40% recurrence rate and 6% mortality!

Bassini, after graduation from medical school, joined the army as a private, to fight in the Italian War of Unification. In combat, he received a bayonet wound to the abdomen, creating a fistula between his intestine and the skin. This was usually a mortal wound. He was treated by Luigi Porta, Chief of Surgery at the University of Padua, Italy. After he recovered, he returned to work as an anatomist and surgeon, serving as Porta's Second Assistant. Much later, he became professor of surgery . He only briefly became involved with hernia surgery, early in a career which included many other areas of endeavor. He advanced hernia surgery in at least four ways, by:

a) Ligating the hernia sac flush with the peritoneum, at the internal ring (other surgeons did not penetrate beyond the external ring)

b) Opening the transversalis fascia, then reconstructing the floor of the inguinal canal

c) Using silk (permanent) sutures, instead of carbolized catgut (which eventually dissolved), and

d) Performing careful audit and follow-up of his patients and their surgical results.

Henry Orlando Marcy, M.D., A.M., L.L.D. (1837-1924), a graduate of Harvard Medical School, was a very unusual physician, for he was independent of universities and clinics. He studied under Lister (who was an orthopedic surgeon) and converted Lister's techniques of antisepsis in orthopedic surgery to allow their use in general and hernia surgery. He described his operation on inguinal hernias at the International Medical Congress in London, in 1881, and Bassini was reputedly in the audience. He described two cases where the internal ring was closed using carbolized sutures or catgut, followed by permanent cure.

Marcy, a talented and industrious man, was also responsible for many important civil engineering projects, including reclaiming the land alongside the Charles River, where M.I.T. is located today.

William Stewart Halsted (1852-1922), was the first professor of surgery at The John Hopkins Medical School. He developed many improved surgical procedures, often based on animal experiments. He was meticulous in his surgical dissection, and was responsible for the development of the "Halstedian school of surgery".

A nurse who worked with him developed eczema from exposure to the harsh chemicals in the operating room. Sympathetic to her plight, he was the first to introduce the use of rubber gloves to be worn in the operating room. He was also the first to study the use of Cocaine as a local anesthetic agent and, unfortunately, became too intimate with its use.

In November, 1889, Dr. Halsted presented five patients on whom he had performed hernia surgery. His method was unique in that Halsted also used the external oblique aponeurosis against the internal oblique muscle, and changed the obliquity of the inguinal canal. Many surgeons, today, feel there is little value in using the external oblique aponeurosis for strength in a hernia repair.

Edward Earle Shouldice (1890-1965), graduated in medicine from the University of Toronto in 1916. He became interested in hernia repairs when treating recruits for military service. Later, Shouldice was appointed lecturer in anatomy at the University of Toronto.

He opened a small, private hospital for the treatment of hernias, using local anesthesia and early ambulation. At first, he used a modified "Bassini repair" and his recurrence rates were high. His associates, N. Obney and E.A. Ryan, studied the Bassini technique being used at the clinic, and redeveloped the original procedure first described by Bassini. Using this "new technique", recurrence rates at the Shouldice Clinic were greatly reduced.

In 1969, the hospital moved to a large, modern facility and over 7,000 hernia repairs are performed there annually.

Amos R. Koontz (1890-1965), had a professional career which spanned the two world wars. Initially trained in biology, he taught at The College of William and Mary for four years, then entered The John Hopkins Medical School in 1914. Planning to graduate in 1918, he joined 31 other volunteers from his class, enlisted into the army as a private. He went overseas with The John Hopkins Hospital Unit Base Hospital #18, where he completed his studies, assisting in the care of war casualties.

In April, 1942, the Hospital Unit was reactivated as the 18th General Hospital under the command of Lt. Col. Amos Koontz, who had enlisted as a private 25 years earlier! His practice and his treatment of war wounds apparently stimulated an interest in abdominal hernias, for he conducted numerous animal experiments and published many articles about the repair of defects of the abdominal wall. He used the patient's own fascia, and substituted inert material, such as Tantalum mesh. As a result of his experimental work and clinical application, he became an international authority on the repair of abdominal hernias. Subsequently, refined synthetic materials, such as Gore-tex® and Marlex®, were developed and have been proven to be well-tolerated by the body as a substitute for living tissue.

Chester Bidwell McVay (1911-1987), was born in Yankton, South Dakota. McVay began his medical school training at Northwestern University. He accepted the challenge of their Honors Program, in which he earned a degree of Doctor of Medicine and also a Doctorate in Anatomy! As a medical student, under the guidance and with with the cooperation of the famous anatomist, Dr. Barry Anson, McVay performed 500 anatomical dissections of the abdominal wall and groin.

He later served as a resident in surgery at the University of Michigan School of Medicine and completed his residency during World War II. His entire resident surgical class was drafted as a unit and sent to Europe. He was in Liege, Belgium, during the Battle of the Bulge, and his unit participated in 16,000 surgical procedures in a period of 15 months during that phase of the war.

Dr. McVay was well regarded for his repair of difficult direct inguinal hernias, with a cure rate of 97%. Because of his contribution, a Cooper's ligament repair is now called a McVay repair.

Summary

The contributions of many gifted men laid the foundation for modern hernia repair. Their tradition of innovation and discovery is carried on today by many fine physicians and surgeons throughout the world. A *few* of the active surgeons who are making significant contributions at this time have been mentioned in this book.

Chapter Seventeen

The Future of Hernia Surgery

Although hernia surgery today offers unprecedented effectiveness, comfort and safety, the future holds promise for even greater improvement on all fronts.

The excellent reputation held by modern medical science is due, in part, to a steadfast adherence to principles of conservatism: no treatment, technique or medication may be introduced without first having passed extensive, calculated tests.

This procedure, or protocol, may be frustrating to the innovative medical scientist, but it is essential to effective care and continued patient confidence.

The emphasis in modern surgery of all types is to reduce the number and size of incisions, to leave as much tissue "untouched" as possible, and to minimize the need for hospitalization.

New Techniques

Among the most exciting surgical techniques for hernia repair now in *experimental* stages is laparoscopic-endoscopic surgical hernia repair. This innovative method has long been in use in other areas of surgery, such as gynecological surgery. Endoscopic procedures currently are being regularly performed in orthopedic surgery of the joints.

In simple terms, endoscopic surgery reduces the size and extent of surgical incisions by allowing the surgeon to work *within* the surgical site while "seeing" the actual surgery via a tiny, highly-mobile television camera. The camera's "eye" is able to penetrate into the surgical site with much less trauma to the area than ordinary methods.

At the present, very few surgeons have experimented with laparoscopic-endoscopic hernia repair. The technique continues to be regarded as controversial, and there have thus far been too few cases to draw any valuable conclusions. Although this form of surgery has been proven successful in reducing hospital time and general discomfort for gallbladder surgery patients, these goals have already been met by conventional hernia surgery techniques. The most important questions remain unanswered: will this exciting new method match the extremely low recurrence rate now enjoyed by conventional hernia surgery patients? If so (and we won't know for about 5 more years), laparoscopic-endoscopic hernia repair surgery may become a viable alternative within the decade.

An equally provocative — and as yet unproven — method may be reconsidered. It may be possible to inject small hernias with a sclerosing agent to "shrink" the hernia sac. Such sclerosing techniques have been very successful in the reduction of varicose veins in the legs. The material injected (a liquid) must be carefully monitored, as earlier experiments did not prove encouraging. Still, new knowledge may shed fresh light on a way to make sclerosing a practical, simple alternative to surgical hernia repair.

About Lasers

Few breakthroughs in medical-surgical care have been greeted with as much public misunderstanding as the laser. Perhaps it was the glamorous treatment of lasers in countless "Star-Wars" and "space" movies. Or maybe the very idea of "surgery" performed with only a barely visible beam of light has captured the public's imagination. Whatever the reason, the public's expectation of the laser's ability has far exceeded its practical application.

Lasers use highly-focused light energy to *cut through* tissue, or to *weld* tissue together. Because the laser light is color sensitive, it can be used to "zap" or quickly remove discolored areas (such as birth marks and pre-cancerous skin lesions) and to close broken blood vessels. The laser beam can pass through the lens of the eye without damage to the lens, then effectively cut or coagulate the deeper layers.

True, the remarkable lasers have proven extremely effective in very *specialized* areas, but as yet have *not* perceivably added either greater success or comfort to hernia surgery.

New types of lasers may hold greater promise of effective application to hernia repair, but are currently extremely experimental in nature.

Hernia Repair in the Fetus

With the advent of *micro*-surgery, the "miniaturization" of surgical techniques opened fascinating possibilities for operating on fetuses *within* the womb. Congenital ("birth") defects may now be repaired prior to birth. A small number of fetuses with congenital diaphragmatic hernias have been successfully operated on using this method. Although currently limited to experimental protocol, such application holds promise for parents and their offspring.

Perhaps even more exciting is the potential for eliminating congenital defects *altogether* through genetic engineering. This "futuristic" technology may someday be used to remove the predisposition to indirect inguinal hernias.

New Materials

Modern hernia repair owes much of its success to the development of marvelous new suturing and strengthening materials. In this area at least, progress continues to be relatively swift and useful.

Mesh and patch materials, used to reinforce repaired areas, will undoubtedly change in shape and texture. Further, meshes are continually being refined relative to fiber type, diameter, nature, size and weave, and size of "interspaces" which allow ingrowth of tissue.

As an example, carbon fiber implants were recently suggested in **Lancet**, a British medical Journal, as a reinforcing material for use in repair of large abdominal wall defects. Carbon fibers are currently being used in orthopedic surgery. They are available in unidirectional, woven or braided form. They are exceptionally strong when first inserted, yet stimulate ingrowth of the body's own dense fibrous tissue which seems to be stronger than the surrounding tissue.

Materials will be developed to hold these meshes in place, perhaps replacing conventional sutures and clips. Dr. René Stoppa, of Ariens, France, has already used a fibrin glue to fasten some of the meshes that he inserts.

Anesthesia

Anesthetic agents and their administration continue to undergo development, evaluation and refinement. "Local" anesthesia has become the method of choice for adult patients, and local anesthesia agents are increasingly stronger, safer and more prolonged. Intravenous general anesthesia now provides *less sedation* and fewer side effects, but greater pain control.

At this time, Patient Controlled Anesthesia, ("PCA") has become increasingly available for hospital and home use. With PCA, patients are able to return home with a computer-controlled injection system which allows pain relief, yet guards against overdose. PCA has been used in the home care of cancer patients and, as its safety is demonstrated, the home use on other patients is being extended.

Costs, Going Up? Going Down?

Cost containment of medical expenses continues to be an ongoing debate. Federally-funded Medicare currently evaluates medical and hospital services and enforces economies. This is a philosophically touchy subject; few people in pain would question the costs for its relief. Yet the very design of modern medical and surgical practice makes some expenses unavoidable. Education, training, equipment and materials — all involve greater sophistication and, therefore, expense.

One idea currently being considered by Medicare is the concept of one all-encompassing payment to a medical team for performance of a particular procedure. Similar to Diagnostic Related Groups ("DRGs") currently used by hospitals for reimbursement, a fixed payment would be divided among all members of the treatment team — irrespective of the number of professionals involved.

As the American population continues to age, and more and more patients turn to Medicare for assistance, it is clear that approved fees for Medicare payment will be reduced.

Summary

The "revolution" in hernia care has produced great benefits to patients today — and will continue to do so in the future.

During the last ten years, enormous strides have been made in the treatment and repair of all types of hernias. As techniques were improved and became less traumatic for the patient, even the aged and medically-compromised could be relieved of the discomfort of hernias.

Patients can look forward to excellent care by highly-trained specialists using the most advanced, proven techniques.

And although the future promises new possibilities, the *present* in hernia treatment truly is "state-of-the-art".

The future of hernia treatment is now!

Glossary

The following are scientific terms used in this book which are defined to enable the lay reader to understand a physician's "jargon". This glossary is prepared, hoping that the reader will more easily comprehend the text.

Acquired hernia - A hernia brought on by lifting or by straining, or by other injury to the tissue, or from degenerative changes of the tissue.

Analgesia - Without the sensation of pain. A condition in which the patient may receive stimuli, but these are not perceived by the patient as painful. Usually accompanied by sedation, but without the loss of consciousness.

Anterior - An anatomical term referring to the front surface of the body. Or, it may refer to the direction toward the front surface, the opposite of "posterior".

Aponeurosis (Plural is aponeuroses) - A fibrous sheet or expanded tendon, giving attachment to the muscular fibers and serving as the means of origin or insertion of a flat muscle.

Atrophy - A wasting of tissues, organs, or the entire body, as from death, disuse, and reabsorption of cells. Diminished cellular volume. Lessened function.

Complete hernia - A type of indirect inguinal hernia in which the contents extend the entire length of the tunica vaginalis. This term is usually used in reference to a male, in which case the hernia extends to the testicle. See figure 4-A, page 33.

Congenital hernia - A hernia which exists at birth, or has the *potential* to exist at birth. It more commonly refers to types of hernias involving the diaphragm or the inguinal area.

Cystocele - A hernia of the bladder into the vaginal wall.

Diaphragmatic hernia - A hernia through the diaphragm. The most common type is the hiatal hernia.

Direct hernia - A type of inguinal hernia. This hernia involves the floor of the inguinal canal.

Double hernia - Two hernias in one area, as contrasted with a bilateral hernia.

Elective - Refers to the performance of a procedure on a scheduled basis, as opposed to an emergency.

Enterocele - A hernial protrusion through a defect in the wall of the vagina between the vagina and the rectum, or between the vagina and bladder. Usually refers to a form of intestinal hernia.

Epigastric hernia - A hernia through the midline of the abdomen, above the umbilicus (navel).

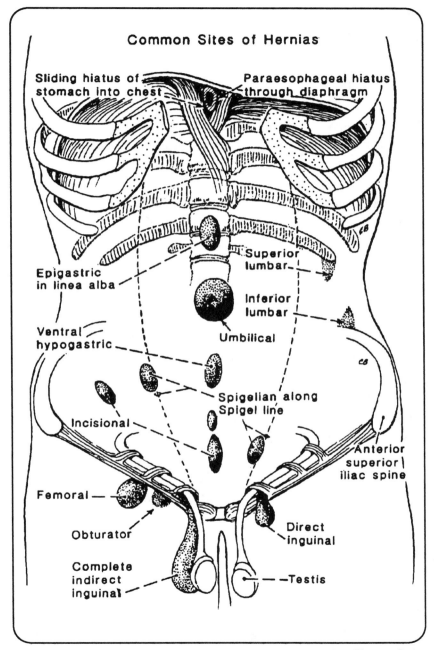

Common Sites of Hernias

Figure G-1

Fascia - A sheet of fibrous tissue that envelops the body beneath the skin. It also encloses muscles and groups of muscles and separates the several layers in groups. In this text, fascia is extended in its use to include some layers of aponeurotic tissue.

Femoral hernia - This is a hernia in the femoral canal, a canal which allows passage of the femoral nerve, artery and vein from pelvis to thigh.

Gangrene - Death of tissue. In reference to hernias, gangrene results from the loss of, or diminution of blood supply to the involved tissue, such as a loop of intestine, because the tissue has been caught and held within a tight ring. Gangrene is frequently associated with bacterial invasion of the involved tissues, with subsequent infection of the area.

Hernia - Rupture. Protrusion of a part or structure through the tissues which normally contain it.

Hydrocele - A collection of serous fluid in a sacculated cavity. Specifically, such a collection in the tunica vaginalis testis, or in a separate pocket along the spermatic cord.

Incarceration - Imprisoned. Constricted. Unnatural retention or confinement of a part. Irreducible. See figure 4-F, page 40

Incisional hernia - A hernia which occurs through a prior abdominal incision.

Incomplete hernia - One which has not passed completely through the orifice or the defect of the wall. This term is often used to describe an inguinal hernia, within the processus vaginalis, but involving only a portion of that potential sac. See figure 4-D, page 37

Inferior - An anatomical term; toward the feet (soles) in relation to another specific point. Opposite of "superior".

Intramuscular hernia - A hernia which lies within the fascial and muscular planes of the abdomen.

Interstitial hernia - The protrusion lies between two of the layers of the abdominal wall, but has not penetrated all of the layers of the muscular wall.

Laparoscopy - To look within the abdominal cavity through a small incision, utilizing an instrument for a direct view, or a miniaturized camera which projects onto a nearby video screen. Performance of this procedure is facilitated by the introduction of gas (CO_2) which distends the abdominal muscles away from the abdominal contents. This allows exposure of some of the organs, and some areas within the abdominal cavity, and some of the abdominal wall.

Lateral - An anatomical term. At or on the side. Further from the midline. Opposite of "medial".

Lineal - Line, in anatomy.

Linea alba - (white line) A fibrous band running vertically in the center of the abdomen. It receives the attachments of the oblique and transverse abdominal muscles. Lying between the rectus muscles, it starts in the upper abdomen at the lower end of the chest and ends at, or just below, the umbilicus.

Lipoma - A fatty accumulation of tissue. A fatty tumor, which is benign. Lipomas occur throughout the subcutaneous tissue of the body and even in the deeper layers, as a usually circumscribed group of mature fat cells. With reference to hernias, fatty tissue tends to accumulate in and alongside the cord structures. This soft tissue may imitate a hernia by pulsating when the patient strains.

Lumbar hernia - A hernia in the back or posterior wall of the abdomen. These are superior, located near the tip of the twelfth rib, and inferior, in the same vertical line, but at the crest of the pelvis.

Medial - An anatomical term, referring to the middle or center of the body, or nearer to that area, as opposed to "lateral".

Mesentery - A double loop of peritoneum attached to the abdominal wall and enclosing in its folds a portion, or all, of the abdominal viscera. The mesentery conveys the vessels and nerves to the viscera.

Neuralgia - Nerve pain. Pain of a throbbing or stabbing character along the distribution of a nerve.

Obturator hernia - A hernia in the pelvic area posterior to the femoral area with protrusion through the obturator foramen, into the deep portion of the thigh.

Oximeter - An instrument for determining photoelectrically the oxygen saturation of a sample of blood, as it courses through the tissues such as an earlobe or fingertip. It constantly monitors and records the patient's oxygen saturation during an operative procedure.

Paraesophageal hernia - A form of hiatal hernia in which a part of the stomach herniates into the chest, but the esophagus remains in its normal position. The result is often a marked distortion of the stomach.

Petit's hernia - A lumbar area hernia on the posterior aspect of the trunk, just superior to the pelvis.

Pneumoperitoneum - The presence of air or gas in the abdominal cavity, or peritoneal cavity. With reference to hernia surgery, this air or gas is introduced artificially to distend the abdominal wall, in preparation for repair of a large hernia. At the time of surgery, the air is released, and the abdominal muscles may then be repaired without tension.

Posterior - An anatomical term. Referring to the back surface of the body or toward the back in reference to another point. Opposite of "anterior", or the front surface of the body.

Present - A common term used by physicians to refer to the appearance of the patient or his illness. To appear for examination. Or, the appearance as seen by the examiner. "The patient presented with—."

Processus vaginalis - A peritoneal diverticulum in the embryonic lower anterior abdominal wall that traverses the inguinal canal. In the male, it forms the tunica vaginalis testis and normally loses its connection with the peritoneal cavity. A persistence of the processus vaginalis in the female is known as the canal of Nuck. See figure 9-C, page 23.

Reducible hernia - One in which the contents may be returned to their normal location by pressure or manipulation.

Richter's hernia - One in which only a part of the wall of an intestinal loop protrudes. This hernia is important because the involved wall of the loop of intestine may be no larger than the fingertip. Diagnosis, therefore, cannot be made on the basis of the size of the protrusion.

Scrotal hernia - An inguinal hernia which has descended into the scrotal sac.

Sliding hernia - A hernia wherein the adjacent organs have "slid" into the hernia sac, and have become a part of that sac. See figure 4-Y, page 59

Spigelian hernia - An abdominal hernia which penetrates just lateral to the strap (rectus) muscles. See Chapter 11, page 140.

Strangulated hernia - A hernia which is tightly constricted and has become, or is likely to become, gangrenous. This is an irreducible hernia, in which the blood circulation may be impeded. Gangrene will occur, unless relief is prompt. See figure 4-F, page 40.

Superior - An anatomical reference; toward the head or top. Opposite of "inferior".

Urethrocele - A hernia of the urethra into the vaginal wall.

Varicocele - A condition manifested by the abnormal dilatation of the veins of the spermatic cord, caused by incompetency of valves in the veins leading to the internal inguinal ring area. This results in a downward influx of blood into the plexus of veins about the cord, when the patient assumes the upright position. Patients often confuse these enlarged veins with a hernia.

Resource material

The interested general and hernia surgeon may wish to have the following list of books and their publishers, for his or her own information. The number of excellent books and atlases published in the past few years indicate the enthusiasm of surgeons for this subject. I find all of them most informative, and would be reluctant to part with any one. Interestingly, the approach by the European authors seem to reflect a very different view of hernia surgery than that of their American counterparts.

The medical journals and articles reviewed for this book were originally listed, and enumerated, but were too extensive and distracted from the flow of the text. An editorial decision was then made to limit the references, hoping that the lay reader would be able to *enjoy* reading the text.

Abdominal Wall Hernias, An Atlas of Anatomy and Repair Madden, John L., W. B. Saunders, 1989

Atlas of Hernia Surgery, Zimmer, Michael, Consulting Editor, B. C. Decker, Inc., 1987

Atlas of Hernia Surgery, Schumpelick, Volker, Verlag, 1987, B. C. Decker, 1990

Atlas of Hernia Surgery, Wantz, George F., Raven Press, 1991

Atlas of Surgical Anatomy for General Surgery, Gray, Steven W., Skandalakis, John F., and McClusky, David A. Illustrated by McClusky, John F., Williams and Wilkins, 1985

Atlas of Topographical and Applied Human Anatomy, Pernkopf, Eduard, Saunders, 1964

Hernia (3rd Edition), Nyhus, Lloyd M., Nyhus and Condon, Lippincott, 1989

HERNIA (Surgical Anatomy and Technique), Skandalakis, John E., Gray, Stephen W., Mansberger, Arlie R. Jr.,Colborn, Gene L., and Skandalakis, Lee J., McGraw Hill, 1989

Hernia Repair Without Disability, Lichtenstein, Irving L., Ishiyoku Euroamerica Inc., 1986

Inguinal Hernia, Nyhus, Lloyd M., Klein, Michael S., and Rogers, Frederick B., Current Problems in Surgery, Mosby-Year Book Inc., June 1991

Management of Abdominal Hernias, Devlin, H. Brendon, Butterworth and Company, 1988

Surgery of the Abdominal Wall, Chevrel, J.P., Springer - Verlag, 1987

Index

A

H

S

T

"A wise person attempts to understand the complexities of the lives of others while reducing ones own life to simplicity."

J.A.B.

"A surgeon is a doctor who can operate and who knows when not to."

Theodore Kocher, (1841-1917)

About the Author,
James A. Bulen, M.D.

Taking time from his hobbies of ceramics, winemaking, and tending his vineyard, Dr. Bulen spent this free time the last year dedicating himself to researching and writing this book. The stimulus for this effort derived from the many questions regarding hernias that he received from his patients and friends in the course of his busy surgical practice in Southern California which emphasizes hernia repair.

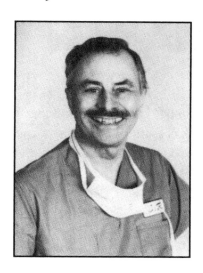

Dr. Bulen received his medical degree from The University of Vermont School of Medicine and his general surgical training at The University of California, San Francisco. He was a flight surgeon in The United States Air Force. Later he returned to Southern California for private practice in general surgery. He is Board Certified in General Surgery and is a Fellow in The American College of Surgeons.

Active in his medical community, Dr. Bulen is a member of The San Diego County Medical Society, serving on the Society's Legislative Committee. He is also a member of the clinical faculty of The University of California, San Diego School of Medicine, participating in the teaching of anatomy to medical students, in their anatomy laboratories.

Dr. Bulen has performed more than 2800 hernia repairs and is currently participating in a hernia research effort at The University of Miami, Miami, Florida.

"It is necessary for a surgeon to have complete, or at least very good, knowledge in anatomy, as well as medicine, so that he has enough judgement and understanding to study all the causes and cicrumstances, and to draw his own conclusions from them."

Lorenz Heister, (1683-1758)

"As long as men are free to ask what they must—free to say what they think—free to think what they will—freedom will never be lost and science can never regress."

J. Robert Oppenheimer, (1904-1967)

About the Illustrator and Co-author, Charles F. Bridgman

A gifted illustrator, Dr. Charles Bridgman has had a distinguished career as Director of the National Medical Audiovisual Center of the National Library of Medicine, and Associate Director of Educational Resources Development. Previously,he was Director of The Office of Learning Resources, University of California, San Diego School of Medicine. He has also taught anatomy and related courses to medical students at both University of California, San Diego and University of California, Los Angeles.

Dr. Bridgman has been a prolific contributor to various biological research papers and articles. His most recent major publication was the text, *Introduction to Functional Histology*, Harper and Row (now Harper and Collins), Publishers, 1990.

Dr. Bridgman lives in La Jolla, California, with his wife, Amy (Ceil), and enjoys his amateur status as an oboeist and English horn player, talents first developed while in high school in Escondido.

He received his undergraduate education at The University of California, Los Angeles and obtained a Certificate in Medical Illustration under Professor Tom Jones at The University of Illinois Medical School. He received a Ph.D. in Anatomical Sciences at The University of California, Los Angeles School of Medicine. His post-doctoral studies were in biomedical communications under David S. Ruhe, M.D., at The University of Kansas Medical Center.

How to buy this book

Telephone orders: Call (619) 746-1123. Have your VISA/Master Card and the following information ready.

Mail orders: Send to: Advanced Health Press, Suite 233-A, 716 East Valley Parkway, Escondido, CA 92025-3097

Fax orders: <u>Fax use is probably the most efficient & economical. Send before 8 a.m. for best rate.</u>

Fax number: (619) 741-1830

Include the following information:

Ship to: _____

Company name: _____

Your Name: _____

Address: _____

City: _____ State: _____ Zip: _____

How to Order:

    ❏ _____ Copies, hard bound, @ $24.95.

    ❏ _____ Copies, soft bound, @ $19.95.

Sales tax: Please add California sales tax if being shipped to CA

Shipping:

    ❏ Book rate: $2.00 for the first book and .75 for each additional book. *(Surface shipping may take three weeks in the U.S.)*

    ❏ Airmail: $3.00 per book.

Payment:

    ❏ Here is my check.

    ❏ My VISA/Master Card number is:

— — — — — — — — — — — — — — — — —

Name on card: _____

Signature _____ Expiration date _____

I understand that I may return this book within 30 days for a full refund, no questions asked.